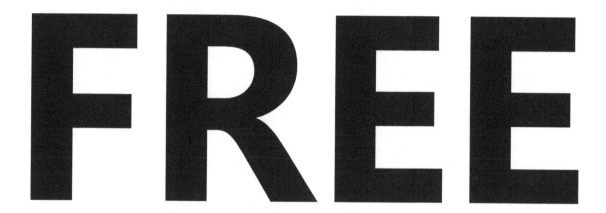

Free Study Tips DVD

In addition to the tips and content in this guide, we have created a FREE DVD with helpful study tips to further assist your exam preparation. **This FREE Study Tips DVD provides you with top-notch tips to conquer your exam and reach your goals.**

Our simple request in exchange for the strategy-packed DVD is that you email us your feedback about our study guide. We would love to hear what you thought about the guide, and we welcome any and all feedback—positive, negative, or neutral. It is our #1 goal to provide you with top quality products and customer service.

To receive your **FREE Study Tips DVD**, email freedvd@apexprep.com. Please put "FREE DVD" in the subject line and put the following in the email:

a. The name of the study guide you purchased.

b. Your rating of the study guide on a scale of 1-5, with 5 being the highest score.

c. Any thoughts or feedback about your study guide.

d. Your first and last name and your mailing address, so we know where to send your free DVD!

Thank you!

CSCS Study Guide 2018 & 2019
CSCS Exam Content & Practice Test Prep Book for the NSCA Certified Strength & Conditioning Specialist Test

APEX Test Prep Personal Trainer Test Prep Team

Table of Contents

Test Taking Strategies

1. Reading the Whole Question

A popular assumption in Western culture is the idea that we don't have enough time for anything. We speed while driving to work, we want to read an assignment for class as quickly as possible, or we want the line in the supermarket to dwindle faster. However, speeding through such events robs us from being able to thoroughly appreciate and understand what's happening around us. While taking a timed test, the feeling one might have while reading a question is to find the correct answer as quickly as possible. Although pace is important, don't let it deter you from reading the whole question. Test writers know how to subtly change a test question toward the end in various ways, such as adding a negative or changing focus. If the question has a passage, carefully read the whole passage as well before moving on to the questions. This will help you process the information in the passage rather than worrying about the questions you've just read and where to find them. A thorough understanding of the passage or question is an important way for test takers to be able to succeed on an exam.

2. Examining Every Answer Choice

Let's say we're at the market buying apples. The first apple we see on top of the heap may *look* like the best apple, but if we turn it over we can see bruising on the skin. We must examine several apples before deciding which apple is the best. Finding the correct answer choice is like finding the best apple. Some exams ask for the *best* answer choice, which means that there are several choices that could be correct, but one choice is always better than the rest. Although it's tempting to choose an answer that seems correct at first without reading the others, it's important to read each answer choice thoroughly before making a final decision on the answer. The aim of a test writer might be to get as close as possible to the correct answer, so watch out for subtle words that may indicate an answer is incorrect. Once the correct answer choice is selected, read the question again and the answer in response to make sure all your bases are covered.

3. Eliminating Wrong Answer Choices

Sometimes we become paralyzed when we are confronted with too many choices. Which frozen yogurt flavor is the tastiest? Which pair of shoes look the best with this outfit? What type of car will fill my needs as a consumer? If you are unsure of which answer would be the best to choose, it may help to use process of elimination. We use "filtering" all the time on sites such as eBay® or Craigslist® to eliminate the ads that are not right for us. We can do the same thing on an exam. Process of elimination is crossing out the answer choices we know for sure are wrong and leaving the ones that might be correct. It may help to cover up the incorrect answer choices with a piece of paper, although if the exam is computer-based, you may have to use your hand or mentally cross out the incorrect answer choices. Covering incorrect choices is a psychological act that alleviates stress due to the brain being exposed to a smaller amount of information. Choosing between two answer choices is much easier than choosing between four or five, and you have a better chance of selecting the correct answer if you have less to focus on.

4. Sticking to the World of the Question

When we are attempting to answer questions, our minds will often wander away from the question and what it is asking. We begin to see answer choices that are true in the real world instead of true in the world of the question. It may be helpful to think of each test question as its own little world. This world may be different from ours. This world may know as a truth that the chicken came before the egg or may

1

assert that two plus two equals five. Remember that, no matter what hypothetical nonsense may be in the question, assume it to be true. If the question states that the chicken came before the egg, then choose your answer based on that truth. Sticking to the world of the question means placing all of our biases and assumptions aside and relying on the question to guide us to the correct answer. If we are simply looking for answers that are correct based on our own judgment, then we may choose incorrectly. Remember an answer that is true does not necessarily answer the question.

5. Key Words

If you come across a complex test question that you have to read over and over again, try pulling out some key words from the question in order to understand what exactly it is asking. Key words may be words that surround the question, such as *main idea, analogous, parallel, resembles, structured,* or *defines*. The question may be asking for the main idea, or it may be asking you to define something. Deconstructing the sentence may also be helpful in making the question simpler before trying to answer it. This means taking the sentence apart and obtaining meaning in pieces, or separating the question from the foundation of the question. For example, let's look at this question:

> Given the author's description of the content of paleontology in the first paragraph, which of the following is most parallel to what it taught?

The question asks which one of the answers most *parallels* the following information: The *description* of paleontology in the first paragraph. The first step would be to see *how* paleontology is described in the first paragraph. Then, we would find an answer choice that parallels that description. The question seems complex at first, but after we deconstruct it, the answer becomes much more attainable.

6. Subtle Negatives

Negative words in question stems will be words such as *not, but, neither,* or *except*. Test writers often use these words in order to trick unsuspecting test takers into selecting the wrong answer—or, at least, to test their reading comprehension of the question. Many exams will feature the negative words in all caps (*which of the following is NOT an example*), but some questions will add the negative word seamlessly into the sentence. The following is an example of a subtle negative used in a question stem:

> According to the passage, which of the following is *not* considered to be an example of paleontology?

If we rush through the exam, we might skip that tiny word, *not,* inside the question, and choose an answer that is opposite of the correct choice. Again, it's important to read the question fully, and double check for any words that may negate the statement in any way.

7. Spotting the Hedges

The word "hedging" refers to language that remains vague or avoids absolute terminology. Absolute terminology consists of words like *always, never, all, every, just, only, none,* and *must*. Hedging refers to words like *seem, tend, might, most, some, sometimes, perhaps, possibly, probability,* and *often*. In some cases, we want to choose answer choices that use hedging and avoid answer choices that use absolute terminology. Of course, this always depends on what subject you are being tested on. Humanities subjects like history and literature will contain hedging, because those subjects often do not have absolute answers. However, science and math may contain absolutes that are necessary for the question to be answered. It's important to pay attention to what subject you are on and adjust your response accordingly.

8. Restating to Understand

Every now and then we come across questions that we don't understand. The language may be too complex, or the question is structured in a way that is meant to confuse the test taker. When you come across a question like this, it may be worth your time to rewrite or restate the question in your own words in order to understand it better. For example, let's look at the following complicated question:

> Which of the following words, if substituted for the word *parochial* in the first paragraph, would LEAST change the meaning of the sentence?

Let's restate the question in order to understand it better. We know that they want the word *parochial* replaced. We also know that this new word would "least" or "not" change the meaning of the sentence. Now let's try the sentence again:

> Which word could we replace with *parochial,* and it would not change the meaning?

Restating it this way, we see that the question is asking for a synonym. Now, let's restate the question so we can answer it better:

> Which word is a synonym for the word *parochial?*

Before we even look at the answer choices, we have a simpler, restated version of a complicated question. Remember that, if you have paper, you can always rewrite the simpler version of the question so as not to forget it.

9. Guessing

When is it okay to guess on an exam? This question depends on the test format of the particular exam you're taking. On some tests, answer choices that are answered incorrectly are penalized. If you know that you are penalized for wrong answer choices, avoid guessing on the test question. If you can narrow the question down to fifty percent by process of elimination, then perhaps it may be worth it to guess between two answer choices. But if you are unsure of the correct answer choice among three or four answers, it may help to leave the question unanswered. Likewise, if the exam you are taking does *not* penalize for wrong answer choices, answer the questions first you know to be true, then go back through and mark an answer choice, even if you do not know the correct answer. This way, you will at least have a one in four chance of getting the answer correct. It may also be helpful to do some research on the exam you plan to take in order to understand how the questions are graded.

10. Avoiding Patterns

One popular myth in grade school relating to standardized testing is that test writers will often put multiple-choice answers in patterns. A runoff example of this kind of thinking is that the most common answer choice is "C," with "B" following close behind. Or, some will advocate certain made-up word patterns that simply do not exist. Test writers do not arrange their correct answer choices in any kind of pattern; their choices are randomized. There may even be times where the correct answer choice will be the same letter for two or three questions in a row, but we have no way of knowing when or if this might happen. Instead of trying to figure out what choice the test writer probably set as being correct, focus on what the *best answer choice* would be out of the answers you are presented with. Use the tips above, general knowledge, and reading comprehension skills in order to best answer the question, rather than looking for patterns that do not exist.

FREE DVD OFFER

Achieving a high score on your exam depends not only on understanding the content, but also on understanding how to apply your knowledge and your command of test taking strategies. **Because your success is our primary goal, we offer a FREE Study Tips DVD, which provides top-notch test taking strategies to help you optimize your testing experience.**

Our simple request in exchange for the strategy-packed DVD is that you email us your feedback about our study guide.

To receive your **FREE Study Tips DVD**, email freedvd@apexprep.com. Please put "FREE DVD" in the subject line and put the following in the email:

    a. The name of the study guide you purchased.

    b. Your rating of the study guide on a scale of 1-5, with 5 being the highest score.

    c. Any thoughts or feedback about your study guide.

    d. Your first and last name and your mailing address, so we know where to send your free DVD!

Introduction to the CSCS Exam

Function of the Test

The CSCS exam is a two-part multiple-choice test required to earn credentials as Certified Strength and Conditioning Specialist (CSCS). These specialists use their training and experience to help safely and effectively improve the athletic performance of athletes of all ages, abilities, and sport goals. The CSCS exam, which is developed and administered by the National Strength and Conditioning Association (NSCA), measures candidates' scientific foundations in exercise sciences and practical applications of strength training and conditioning knowledge and skills.

Candidates interested in taking the CSCS must demonstrate their fulfillment of the eligibility criteria by submitting the appropriate documentation within one year after the date they took the exam. Exam results are voided if the eligibility documentation is not received within this timeframe. To be eligible for the exam, candidates must hold at least a bachelor's degree from an accredited institution or be currently enrolled as a college senior such an institution. A list of the six accepted regional accrediting associations is available on the NSCA website (https://www.nsca.com/cscs-exam-prerequisites/). Candidates must provide proof of their academic eligibility by sending an official transcript from an institution accredited by one of the six associations. A similar educational level or degree must be achieved by candidates residing outside of the United States and Canada. Note that test takers who take the test during their senior year of college are not certified immediately upon passing the exam. Instead, certification is granted once they have successfully graduated college and the NSCA has received their official transcript confirming their degree completion. All candidates must also hold a current CPR and AED certification from a course that has a hands-on, in-person component and requires an evaluation of skills. Therefore, courses that are completed entirely online or that only involve a written exam are not acceptable. If the candidate has an expired CPR/AED certification or has not yet earned certification, he or she must obtain certification and mail the NSCA proof within one calendar year of the exam date. Even after successfully passing the exam, CSCS certification will not be granted to a candidate until the NSCA has received verification of all eligibility requirements.

Candidates sitting for the CSCS usually have an educational background and/or professional experience in exercise science/physiology, kinesiology and biomechanics, strength training and conditioning, or physical therapy and athletic training. According to the NSCA, in 2017, the pass rate for the CSCS exam was 53%.

Test Administration

Throughout the year, CSCS exams are offered worldwide at Pearson VUE test locations. NSCA members can take the exam for a lower fee than non-members, though membership is not required for certification. Both sections of the CSCS (Scientific Foundations and Practical/Applied) must be taken by candidates who are sitting for the exam for the first time. A passing grade is needed on both sections to receive CSCS credentials. If a test taker achieves a passing score on just one of the two sections, he or she may retake just the failed section on subsequent attempts. A candidate may retake both or just one section of the CSCS as many times as he or she desires, although a waiting period of 90 days follows each attempt, during which the candidate may not yet register. After this time has elapsed, the candidate can retake the exam. Candidates needing accommodations for documented disabilities may make such arrangements with the Pearson VUE testing center directly.

Test Format

The CSCS exam consists of two sections. The first section, Scientific Foundations, lasts 1.5 hours and contains 80 scored and 15 unscored multiple-choice questions that address exercise sciences and nutrition. The Practical/Applied section, which lasts 2.5 hours, contains 110 scored and 15 unscored multiple-choice questions that address program design, exercise technique, testing and evaluation, and organization/administration. Approximately 30-40 questions in this section contain videos and/or images; these, and other questions, may assess competencies across multiple domains simultaneously.

The breakdown of the Scientific Foundations section, including example topics for each subsection, is as follows:

Field	Percent of Section	Number of Questions
Exercise Sciences (Anatomy and Physiology, Physiological Adaptations to Exercise, Biomechanics, Bioenergetics, Psychological Techniques, Physiological Differences Between Athletes)	74%	59
Nutrition (Effects of Nutrition on Health and Performance, Food Choices to Maximize Performance, Eating Disorders, Ergogenic Aids)	26%	21
Unscored Questions		15
Total	**100%**	**95**

The breakdown of the Practical/Applied section, including example topics for each subsection, is as follows:

Field	Percent of Section	Number of Questions
Exercise Technique (Resistance Training, Plyometrics, Agility, Flexibility, etc., and Spotting)	35%	38
Program Design (Training Methods and Modes, Exercise Selection and Order, Volume and Intensity, Progression, Recovery, Periodization)	35%	39
Organization and Administration (Design and Layout of Strength Training Facilities, Duties and Responsibilities, Policies, Ensuring a Safe Training Environment)	12%	13
Testing and Evaluation (Selecting and Administering Tests, Testing Procedures, Interpreting Results)	18%	20
Non-scored Questions		15
Total	**100%**	**125**

Test takers are given a break between the two sections, which is not included in the times listed for each section. The unscored questions are mixed randomly throughout the exam so that test takers are unaware of which questions count towards their score and which do not. The test developers use the unscored questions as "pretest" questions for consideration as potential scored questions on future exams. As they are unscored, these questions do not affect a test taker's final score or impact his or her pail/fail status.

Scoring

Each of the two sections of the CSCS exam is scored on a scale ranging from 1 to 99. Candidates must earn at least a 70 on each section to attain passing status. These scaled scores are calculated from the raw scores using different formulas and metrics that take into account the difficulty of each question. The scaling process allows scores to be compared across various versions of the test and years of administration. Therefore, a scaled score of 82 earned by a test taker in 2017 is equivalent to a scaled score of 82 achieved by a test taker in 2016.

Exercise Sciences

One of the main roles of a strength and conditioning professional is to apply foundation knowledge in program design and administration. Therefore, it is vitally important to acquire a thorough understanding of the human body and all the intricate systems that apply to the physical preparation of human performance. By acquiring this knowledge, the strength and conditioning professional can ensure that the training of athletes is performed in a safe and effective manner and that specific adaptions are occurring in conjunction with the sporting demands.

Muscle Anatomy and Physiology

The musculoskeletal system contains all the muscles that comprise the axial skeleton and the appendicular skeleton. The *axial skeleton* consists of the ribs, sternum, vertebral column, and the skull and the *appendicular skeleton* includes the bones of the hips, knees, ankles, feet, pelvic girdle, shoulder girdle, arms, wrists, and hands. Each one of these bones are connected by joints. Different types of joints include fibrous joints, such as those in the skull, cartilaginous joints, like those between vertebrae, and synovial joints, such as those in the shoulder and hip. Each of the theses bones and joints are able to move via the musculature of the human body.

Muscle Anatomy

The strength and conditioning professional must first be able to identify and target each muscle group within the human body. It is vitally important to understand the correct terminology and location of muscles as well as the movements they allow to offer safe, effective training to athletes, and also to communicate appropriately when collaborating with the athletic training staff and team doctors for rehabilitation purposes.

The above illustration is a great resource for most of the specific names of the major skeletal muscles. Along with the specific names of the muscles, the strength and conditioning professional should also possess an understanding on the main muscle groups of the body and to which of these groups each specific muscle belongs. The major muscle groups of the human body consist of the calves, hamstrings, quadriceps, glutes, abdominals, pecs, latissimus dorsi, trapezius, biceps, triceps, and muscles of the forearms. Having a thorough understanding of each of the actions of these muscle groups will enhance the ability to discuss training programs, design effective periodization plans, understand rehabilitation protocols, and program return to play for athletes. Once a basic understanding is attained, the strength and conditioning professional can move deeper into the fundamental structures of each muscle fiber.

Most bones are surrounded by a specialized tissue called bone *periosteum.* The bone periosteum is the area of bone which connects the bone to muscle via tendons. The location of where a muscle connects to bone is also important to understand. For muscles of the limbs, the attachment that is typically proximal (closer to the trunk) is termed the *origin,* while the attachment that is usually more distal (further from the trunk down the extremity) is termed the *insertion.* For muscles of the trunk, the origin is usually more superior (closer to the head), and the insertion is more inferior (towards the feet).

Each of the muscles of the human body will have common characteristics. The cells of the musculature system are called *muscle fibers* and are surrounded by connective tissues that keep them in respective bundles. First, the *epimysium* consists of the connective tissue that surrounds the outermost surface area of each skeletal muscle. Going further inward, under the epimysium, individual muscle fibers are bundled into groups called *fascicles*, which are coated by the covering called *perimysium*. Fascicles can contain many fibers and can even have up to 150 muscle fibers contained within the bundle. Even deeper within, the *endomysium* surrounds each individual muscle fiber within the fascicle. The connective tissues of the epimysium, perimysium, and endomysium are connected to the tendons of the body so that any tension of the muscles can be translated to the tendons and therefore, pull on the bones, causing movement of the body.

Major Skeletal Muscles of the Human Body

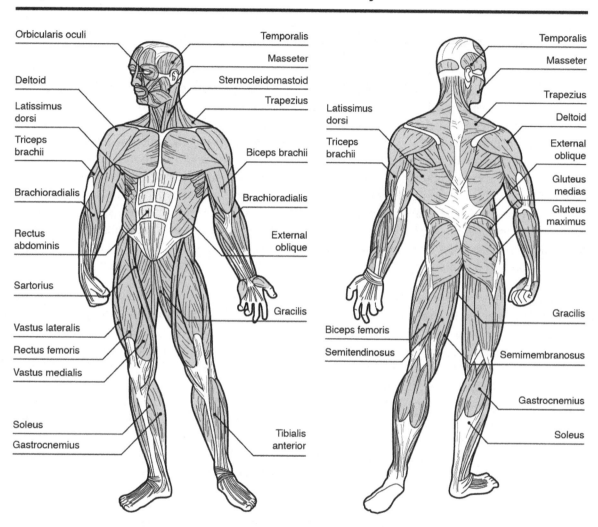

To initiate the muscular contractions that cause movement, an excitation (stimulus) from a nerve cell travels to the muscle fibers. This nerve cell is referred to as a *motor neuron* and can be responsible for movement for up to several hundred muscle fibers. The *motor unit* is the term used for the motor neuron and the skeletal muscle fibers that specific neuron innervates. The *axon* is at proximal end of the motor neuron. The portion between the axonal terminals and the muscle fibers is called the neuromuscular junction and once the signal jumps from the motor neuron to the muscle fibers, the muscle will now contract, causing movement. Each muscle fiber is only innervated by one motor neuron, though each motor neuron can have anywhere from several to several thousand skeletal muscle fibers associated with it.

Within each single muscle fiber are *myofibrils*. These myofibrils contain two different *myofilaments* that are directly responsible for the contraction of the muscle. The thicker filament is called *myosin* and the thinner one is *actin*. Myosin filaments are characterized by a globular head and a movable hinge. The actin filaments are characterized by two strands in a double helix. The globular head of the myosin interacts with the double helix of the actin and this interaction is called a *cross-bridge*. The movement of the globular head pulling and releasing along the actin's double helix is what causes movement within the muscle fiber.

Muscular Dynamics Involved During Movement Patterns

In simple terms, the sliding-filament theory states that actin and myosin filaments interact with each other by binding, pulling, and sliding. To begin understanding this concept, some basic terminology of the components involved must be learned. The *sarcomere* is the functional contractile unit of a muscle fiber. Within the sarcomere is where the myosin and actin filaments are located. When looking at the sarcomere from a cross-sectional view, the *m-bridge* or m-line is a dark colored band where two adjacent myosin filaments are connected. Across the m-bridge and on the opposite end of the sarcomere is the *z-line*. Each sarcomere is defined by the z-lines such that a sarcomere begins at one z-line and ends at another (and another starts there and ends at the next). The z-line is the location where actin filaments are anchored. When still looking at a sarcomere from a cross-sectional view there are also other areas; the A-band, the I-band, and the H-zone. The A-*band* is the area of the sarcomere that bookends each myosin filament. The *I-band* is the area of the sarcomere that contains only actin filaments. Lastly, the *H-zone* is the center area of the sarcomere that contains only myosin filaments with no overlapping actin.

The sliding-filament theory has the actin moving through the sarcomere thus moving the ends (Z-lines) towards each other as the muscle fiber shortens. While the actin filaments are interacting with the myosin filaments, the H-zone and I-band will shrink as the Z-line starts moving towards each other. During actin and myosin filament interaction, calcium must be present for the binding and sliding (and thus contraction) to occur. When the muscle is at rest, most of the calcium is stored in the sarcoplasmic reticulum; therefore, little interaction is happening during the resting phase. This initial interaction will then start to begin during the excitation-contraction coupling phase. During this portion of the sliding-filament theory, calcium is released and binds to *troponin*, a protein that is embedded with the actin filament. Once calcium binds to troponin, a counteraction occurs in *tropomyosin*, which also is contained within the double helix of the actin filament. This counteraction will cause the actin to become pulled towards the center of the sarcomere, exposing more potential binding sites for the myosin heads to attach.

After the excitation-contraction coupling phase is the contraction phase. During the contraction phase, adenosine triphosphate (ATP), the energy molecule of the cell, is broken down into adenosine diphosphate (ADP). After this breakdown, another phosphate group needs to be added to ADP for the globular myosin head to break free of the actin filament. Without another phosphate group added, and as long as calcium is available, the myosin and actin will stay in contact with each other. Therefore, it can be concluded that ATP and calcium are required for interaction between actin and myosin. Following the contraction phase is the recharge phase. Contraction is continued during the recharge phase and many of the same components of the contraction phase continue to occur during the recharge phase: calcium connecting to troponin, actin beginning to interact with myosin, dissociation of actin to myosin, and lastly, the myosin head recharging to again come in contact with actin.

Once the muscle receives a signal to relax (either from lack of calcium or stoppage from the motor nerve), the actin and myosin will be prevented from interacting with each other. Calcium, or lack thereof, plays a major role in the relaxation phase. Whether there is a low supply of calcium or the motor nerve stops sending a signal, the calcium will go back into the sarcoplasmic reticulum and can no longer be used for the actin and myosin filament cross-bridge. When the actin and myosin filaments can no longer interact, the muscle will relax.

Neuromuscular Anatomy and Physiology

Neuromuscular Anatomy

The motor neurons and the muscle cells they innervate make up the neuromuscular system. The electrical impulse that is sent through the spinal cord to the axon, down the axon terminal, and into the muscle is called the *action potential*. This action potential does not have full capability to contract muscles but instead, it signals other actions to occur for the contraction of muscle. It is important to note that some motor neurons innervate many muscle fibers and some motor neurons innervate very few fibers. The motor neurons that innervate many muscle fibers are primarily responsible for large muscle actions such as those in the quadriceps group or gastrocnemius. The motor neurons that only innervate a few muscle fibers are responsible for more precise movements, such as those in the eye or fingers.

Once the action potential has been sent down the axon terminal, it will arrive at the *nerve terminal*. It is here that the chemical reaction responsible for direct muscle contraction occurs. Once the action potential reaches the nerve terminal, a release of *acetylcholine* occurs. Acetylcholine then travels to the neuromuscular junction and causes a reaction of the sarcolemma. Acetylcholine will then create a "bridge" to where the action potential can transfer into the muscle. As long as the action potential stimulus that reaches the sarcolemma exceeds a certain threshold, all of the fibers in the motor unit will contract. This is known as the all-or-none principle. Essentially, so long as the stimulus exceeds the threshold, all the muscle fibers were fire and contract and if the stimulus fails to reach the threshold, none of the fibers in the motor unit will contract. There is no partial contraction whereby only some fibers contract.

Understanding of the muscle fiber types is important for the strength and conditioning professional. These fiber types play a role in training responses as well as metabolic demands in athletic preparation. The two main muscle fiber types are fast-twitch fibers and slow-twitch fibers. As the name suggests, each fiber type is classified based on the twitch time the muscle fiber requires. All muscle fibers that are innervated within a motor neuron consist of the same fiber type. Therefore, a fast-twitch motor unit will consist of all fast-twitch muscle fibers and a slow-twitch motor unit will consist of all slow-twitch muscle fibers. Fast-twitch muscle fibers are powerful fibers that fatigue quickly but can produce contraction and relaxation quickly. Slow-twitch muscle fibers will require more time for contraction and relaxation, but their endurance is greater. Under magnification, each fiber can also fall into more specific classifications; Type I, Type II, and Type IIx. Type I fibers are classified as slow-twitch muscle fibers. Type II and Type IIx are both fast-twitch muscle fibers. The main difference between Type II fibers (also classified as Type IIa) and Type IIx is their ability to use aerobic-oxidative energy as a fuel source. Type IIa fibers contain more mitochondria and therefore, they can produce energy aerobically more than Type IIx can. The following lists provide the basic characteristics of each fiber type:

Type I
- Efficient muscle fibers
- Slow to fatigue
- High mitochondrial density

- Low anaerobic power
- Lack ability for powerful contractions

Type II (Type IIa)
- Less efficient
- Easily fatigued
- Low aerobic power
- Ability to contract rapidly
- Moderate mitochondrial density

Type IIx
- Least efficient
- Easiest to fatigue
- Most powerful
- Highest anaerobic power

There are various specialized sensory receptors located among the muscle fibers. These sensory receptors are termed *proprioceptors*. Proprioceptors are located among muscles, joints, and tendons and relay spatial awareness to the conscious and subconscious of the human body. Two of the main proprioceptors that the strength and conditioning professional must be aware of are the Golgi tendon organs (GTOs) and muscle spindles. GTOs are proprioceptors located in the tendons of the human body. These proprioceptors become active when the tendon stretches. As the tendon stretches beyond normal limits and tension increases within the muscle, the GTO will inhibit the muscle of contraction, decreasing the likelihood of injury. Just as a motor neuron controls the signal to the muscle, GTO's have a sensory neuron that relays information to and from the nervous system. Most of the activity of GTOs comes from heavy resistance in training and their reactive ability can be trained through a progressive training program.

Muscle spindles, another type of proprioceptor, are specialized muscle fibers located within the connective tissue. These specialized muscle fibers run parallel to the normal muscle fibers, but instead of being controlled by a motor neuron, they are controlled by a sensory neuron that relays messages back to the nervous system. Muscle spindles primarily work by relaying information on the length of the muscle and the rate of change in the length. When the muscle lengthens, or quickly changes length, the muscle spindles are stretched, and they relay a message to the spinal cord that a potentially dangerous stretch is occurring. This signal then connects with the efferent signal of the motor neuron and either causes the contraction to cease (to prevent damage) if the stretch is too great, or permits the contraction. A common example of this proprioceptor is the knee-jerk reaction. When the patellar tendon is tapped, the muscle spindles of the knee extensors are stretched, and a signal is relayed to spinal cord, telling the muscles of the knee extensors to activate.

Neuromuscular Responses to Exercise

It is important for the strength and conditioning professional to understand the responses of the neuromuscular system to exercise. Having a thorough understanding of how to body responds to the physical stress of training will allow the strength and conditioning professional to program the training based on the scientific foundations of exercise.

Every time a sufficiently-strong action potential travels down the axon terminal, a short activation occurs in the muscle fibers. This short activation is termed a *twitch*. If a second twitch occurs before the first twitch completely relaxes, the twitches will overlap and create a stronger muscle contraction. The overlapping of two or more twitches is termed *summation*. If twitches continue to occur prior to the previous twitches relaxing, a total contraction, called *tetanus*, is possible within the muscle fibers.

During training, as well as during normal activities, the body has the ability to control the output of the muscles for certain tasks. The force needed to pick up a piece of paper from the ground is different than the force of a maximal deadlift, although both activities are using the same movement patterns. The ability to control the force output of muscles can be accomplished in two ways. The first is the recurrence of activation of the motor units. If the motor unit is only activated once, such as in a twitch, the force will be low for that given muscle group. However, as twitches begin to overlap and summate, the force developed will become more powerful than that of a single twitch. The second way the body has the ability to control the force of the output is through changing the number of motor units activated. The process in which the body selects the number of motor units activated is termed *recruitment*. During recruitment, the body can determine how many motor units are required for a given activity, as well as what type of fibers are needed for the activity. For the near maximal deadlift, the body would primarily use Type IIx fibers since they can generate the most force in the shortest amount of time. Since the maximal deadlift attempt should not take longer than ten seconds, the body is not concerned with the aerobic capacity of the muscle fiber. If the athlete were to be running a marathon, the type and number of muscle fibers activated would differ. For a marathon runner, the body would prioritize Type I fibers since they are much more resistant to fatigue.

Basic Principles of Biomechanics

Acquiring a basic understanding of biomechanics will greatly enhance the effectiveness of the strength and conditioning professional. The understanding of basic biomechanics can help identify sport performance needs of the athlete and enhance the effectiveness of the training program. *Biomechanics* is the term for the mechanics of the musculoskeletal system as it relates to human movement.

Kinematic Principles of Movement

When designing programs for specific sporting activities, it is helpful to understand where the majority of the movement within the sport is taking place. These locations occur within the sagittal plane, the frontal plane, or the transverse plane. These terms relate to movements occurring when viewing the human body in the anatomical position: standing erect with the arms down, palms facing forward, head looking straight ahead, and the feet flat on the ground. The *sagittal plane* is the plane where movement takes place in a forward or backward motion. The sagittal plane would be a plane splitting the anatomical position directly down center and creating left and right halves. The *frontal plane* is where movement takes place in a lateral, side to side, motion. The frontal plane would consist of a plane splitting the anatomical position into anterior and posterior halves. Lastly, the *transverse plane* is the plane where movement takes place in a rotational motion parallel to the ground. The transverse plane would consist of a plane splitting the body in the anatomical position into top and bottom halves, usually around the naval.

The following provide an example of the hip joint moving in each of the planes:

- *Sagittal Plane Movement*: Flexion and Extension
- *Frontal Plane Movement*: Adduction and Abduction
- *Transverse Plane Movement*: Internal Rotation and External Rotation

Body Planes

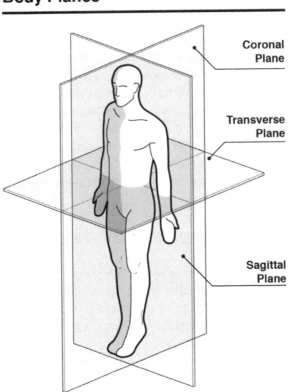

While the human body is moving through each plane, it is important to note how joint angles play a role in attaining proper biomechanics. As the body moves through the full range of motion, more force is needed throughout to counteract the forces within each portion of the movement. The *moment arm* is the term used for the distance from the line of action of the force to that of the pivot point of the joint. When the moment arm is longer, there is more of a mechanical advantage because the lever length is effectively increased, and when the moment arm is shorter, the potential torque using the same force is less because the lever length is shorter (note: torque is force multiplied by the moment arm). Taking the biceps curl as an example, the moment arm is at a mechanical disadvantage when the weight is held in the lower position. Understanding mechanical advantage and disadvantage can enhance the effectiveness in exercise selection throughout the training cycle.

Another area of consideration that must be addressed is that of the velocity of the muscle contraction. During the contraction of the muscle, the higher the velocity, the lower the force capability. Therefore, subconscious, normal biomechanics of the human body will tend to attempt to slow the velocity down to try to increase the force of the muscles being activated. A common example of this is the arm action of a vertical jump. As the arms move downward, lower velocities are capable since more force than just the body is being applied to the body. It is here that the knees and hips can contract with more force allowing the body to apply more force for the jump.

14

Kinetic Laws and Principles of Movement

It is important for the strength and conditioning professional to understand the basic kinematic laws and principles of movement. These laws and principles will provide an understanding of the force required for all athletic movements.

To begin, it is important to understand basic terminology in the kinetic laws and principles of movement. *Momentum* is the term used to define the correlation between mass and the velocity of movement of that mass. As a mass increases its velocity, more force will be required to change the direction of movement due to the increased momentum in the initial certain direction. The *fulcrum* is the main pivot point of a lever and *torque* is considered the degree at which the force rotates around the fulcrum. When analyzing actual positive work and power as it pertains to human movement, *power* is defined as the rate at which the work is performed, where work is the force applied in a particular direction and the displacement of the object due to the force being applied. The force can be considered the push or pull applied to an object, which can also be the human body, which separates the two objects from one another. With this knowledge, the strength and conditioning professional can now understand the basic equations for positive work and power of the human body. *Work*, when viewed as a simple equation, is force multiplied by displacement. Once work is determined, power can be defined through another equation. *Power* is calculated as work divided by time.

Laws of Kinetics
Moving into more advanced principles and laws of kinetics, the strength and conditioning professional must understand particular terms of physics as they relate to specific movements of the human body. *center of gravity* is the location at which the body will remain in balance. This location will allow the object to stay in balance when external forces are placed upon the object. Taller athletes, therefore, have a higher center of gravity than do shorter athletes. One's center of gravity is lowered as the body is lowered, for example in a deep squat, and this generally affords an easier ability to balance. An *impulse* is the ability for an object to change its location by applying force to produce a change in velocity. The impulse considers the force applied as well as the length of time over which the force is applied. This pressure that is being applied will also have a center of gravity in a specific location. The center of gravity at which the pressure is being applied is termed the *center of pressure*.

Muscle Action
Another area in which the strength and conditioning professional must be proficient is that of muscle action, called *contractions*. Muscle action of the human body is primarily described as three different actions: concentric contractions, eccentric contractions, and isometric contractions. Concentric contractions shorten the length of the muscle. This contraction is due to the actin and myosin interacting with each other. The force that is created from the concentric muscle action is greater than that of the external resistance; therefore, shortening of the musculature occurs during movement. Eccentric muscle action occurs when the muscle is lengthened due to the external force acting upon it. The force that is created from eccentric muscle action is less than that of the external force; therefore, lengthening of the musculature occurs. Concentric muscle action and eccentric muscle action have a paired relationship with one another and many exercises use both muscle actions. Using a biceps curl as an example, bringing the weight up from the arms in a straightened position to one where the elbows are bent is a concentric contraction. Straightening the elbows back out and lowering the weight involves an eccentric contraction of the biceps. During isometric muscle action the length of the muscles involved in movement do not change. During isometric contractions, the force of the musculature and external resistance is equal to one another. Using the curl as an example again, after the weight reaches the uppermost part of the movement (elbows fully bent) and before it reverses direction to be lowered, there is a slight pause where

the load and contractile force are equal. It is during this portion of the exercise that isometric muscle action occurs.

Levers

Movement of the human body comes from contraction of muscles pulling on joints. As described previously, these joints move around the fulcrum and on the levers formed by bones. These levers are classified as first-, second-, or third-class levers. A first-class lever is one in which the fulcrum is between muscular force and the external resistance (the load). An example of a first-class lever in human movement is the head moving on the neck such that the chin touches the chest or one looks up at the sky. A second-class lever is one in which the external resistance (the load) is between the fulcrum and the muscular force. A common example of an exercise that uses a second-class lever is that of a calf raise, since the calves and external resistance (human body plus external resistance) act on the same side to raise the heel from the ground as in plantar flexion. Lastly, a third-class lever is one in which the muscular force is between the fulcrum and the load. A common example of an exercise that uses a third-class lever for movement is that of a bicep curl since the biceps and brachialis work on the same side as the external resistance of the barbell or dumbbell.

Roles of Muscles in Movement

As previously stated, muscles are attached to bone by tendons. As the contraction of the muscle occurs, the shortening of the muscle pulls on the bone and causes movement. The muscle that's involved in the contraction is known as the *agonist* and is considered the *prime mover* of the movement. The *antagonist*, which is the muscle involved in slowing down the contraction or stopping the movement, elongates as the agonist is contracting. For every main movement of the human body, there will be an agonist and an antagonist muscle or muscles. Within movement, there is also another category of muscle involvement called synergists. *Synergists* are muscles that are not directly involved with the movement but assist in stabilization of the joints. Lastly, *neutralizers* are muscles that act as agonists but do not move. Neutralizers are agonists in terms of stabilization, but instead of contracting as a prime mover would, they instead prevent movement from forces being applied from the external resistance. For the strength and conditioning professional, having a thorough understanding of all the muscle movements and contributions involved in a single movement is critical for optimal training. The strength and conditioning professional should acquire the ability to term each agonist, antagonist, synergist, and neutralizer muscle within each movement used in the training program.

Bone and Connective Tissue Anatomy and Physiology

Bone and Connective Tissue Anatomy

Acquiring a basic knowledge of bone and connective tissue anatomy can enhance the understanding of the adaptations that occur to these structures during athletic training. Basic bone anatomy consists of non-living mineral components as well as living bone cells. Bone is primarily made of calcium carbonate, calcium phosphate, and collagen, which is a protein. As previously described, bone periosteum makes up the outer layer of bone and serves as an attachment point for connective tissues. Underneath the periosteum is the bone itself. Bone consists of a hard outer layer of compact mineralized substances that are supported by strong collagen fibers. The compact outer layer is also known as *cortical* bone. The outer layer also consists of osteocytes, which are bone cells. *Trabecular* bone lies underneath the cortical bone. Trabecular bone refers to the spongy bone that is located within the cortical bone. This spongy area allows for the bone to be light from the spongy spaces but strong enough to withstand forces. Trabecular bone tends to develop into specific open areas that consist of bone marrow and the trabeculae arrange themselves in response to the stresses placed on the bone.

All joints of the human body contain tendons and ligaments that provide stability throughout movement. These ligaments consist of a collagen bundle that encases the connective fibers that enclose the fibrils and microfibrils. Collagen is the main substance in all connective tissue. Collagen fibers, much like muscle fibers, consist of Type I and Type II fibers. Type I fibers primarily compose tendons and ligaments and Type II fibers are primarily in cartilage.

Bone and Connective Tissue Responses to Exercise and Training

Just as the musculature of the human body responds to training, bone and connective tissue do as well. To withstand the forces that can occur from training, bone and connective tissue must also adapt. Training programs can enhance these adaptations to the bone and connective tissue. The strength and conditioning professional must acquire knowledge of certain training parameters that can enhance these adaptations.

Adaptations that occur to the bones often occur from forces placed upon them from external resistance. The osteocytes of the bone include *osteoblasts* that can form and produce new bone growth. During non-training periods, these osteoblasts are dormant. During training periods when forces are placed on the bones, the osteoblasts become active, migrating towards the bones regions where stresses are experiences where they will begin bone remodeling. This migration process will end at the portion of the bone that encounters the most force, usually within the center of the bone. After migration occurs, new bone formation will begin. Bone formation occurs as new collagen fibers are laid on stressed sites. Mineralization of the collagen fibers then makes the bone stronger and able to withstand higher forces.

For the strength and conditioning professional, it is important to understand which modalities are optimal for the stimulation of bone formation. For new bone formation, isolated exercises should be used sparingly. Isolation exercises do not have the ability to apply the amount of stress needed for formation of new bone. Therefore, when formation of new bone is desired, the strength and conditioning professional should select exercises that are ground-based, multi-joint movements. Also, movements that load the spine through movements of the hips, knees, and ankles tend to produce more formation of new bone than other exercises. Beyond external resistance, the strength and conditioning professional can also choose exercises that place high forces on the body via high-intensity impact movements. Examples of weight-bearing exercises that don't include additional resistance in the form of weights are plyometric exercises and sprinting. Both of these types of exercises place tremendous loads the body and have the potential to stimulate new bone formation.

Since the musculature and bone both adapt to external resistance, the tendons and ligaments of the body must do the same to withstand the loads that the muscle and bone can now produce. The tendons and ligaments of the human body increase their ability to withstand force by multiple means. The following are examples of ways that tendons and ligaments adapt to withstand forces from training:

- The diameter of the fibrils increases
- Cross-links occur at higher rates (density increases)
- New collagen fibers develop, increasing the number of connective fibers

For the strength and conditioning professional, it is important to understand what training variables can be incorporated to increase the adaptations of connective tissue. Many of the movements that are required for new bone formation can also be used to stimulate connective tissue adaptations, as long as the movements are performed with special attention on certain aspects of the exercise. Ground-based, multi-joint movements that are used to drive new bone formation can also require adaptation from tendons and ligaments as long as intensities remain high and full range of motion occurs on every repetition. It is important to note that adaptations of connective tissue do not occur at moderate or low intensities. Therefore, higher intensities are required if adaptations of connective tissue are desired.

Bioenergetics and Metabolism

Characteristics of the Energy Systems

Understanding the biological energy systems of the human body is vitally important for the strength and conditioning professional. Being able to differentiate the characteristics of each of the metabolic energy systems, as well as how to develop these systems, is a major component of the strength and conditioning profession. First and foremost, the strength and conditioning professional must understand the energy being used for different sporting activities. Sporting specificity as it relates to conditioning is critical in developing the primary and secondary energy systems used for the activity.

The energy molecule adenosine triphosphate (ATP) is the fuel source that drives all muscle action. All energy for movement of the human body is caused when ATP cleaves off one phosphate group and becomes adenosine diphosphate (ADP). This reaction releases energy that can be harnessed to do muscular work. To replenish ATP from ADP, a reaction must occur to regain the phosphate group that was removed. This replenishment will be acquired from one of the three biological energy systems of the human body. The energy systems of the human body consist of the phosphagen system, the glycolytic system, and the oxidative system. Each one of these energy systems will replenish ATP though the rate, location within the cell, and pathway through which ATP is replenished differentiates the systems. During sporting activities, the human body will often use each of these systems simultaneously, but the rate and degree of reliance on each system is dependent on the intensity, effort, and duration of the activity.

The phosphagen and glycolytic biological energy systems are anaerobic energy systems. Therefore, they do not require oxygen for their reactions. The *phosphagen system* is the primary energy system used in the beginning of movement. Since the phosphagen system is the first source of ATP, the ATP is readily available, and the body will use the ATP from the phosphagen system at the onset of any activity. The shortcoming of the phosphagen system is that the ATP available via this system will only fuel high-intensity activities lasting approximately 10 seconds or less. Activities that primarily use the phosphagen system as fuel are exercises that consist of short duration and high intensity. Examples include short sprints at full speed, shot put, Olympic lifting, and throwing a baseball with maximal force. Once the ATP production of the system starts to deplete, the body will start working to produce energy via the glycolytic system.

The *glycolytic energy system*, also called glycolysis, is considered the primary energy system used for activities lasting 10 seconds to 2-3 minutes. This system can also be broken down into two subgroups: fast glycolysis and slow glycolysis. Glycolysis produces *pyruvate* as an end result and the fate of that molecule determines which subgroup proceeds. When pyruvate is converted to lactate, ATP will replenish at a fast rate and therefore, it will be available for fuel. Unfortunately, this fuel will only last a short time before the energy demands will need to be met from another source. Fast glycolysis tends to only produce energy for approximately 15-30 seconds before the body will begin to rely on slow glycolysis. Slow glycolysis occurs when pyruvate is not converted into lactate but instead enters the Krebs cycle. The replenishment of ATP will occur at a slower rate, though it will be able to fuel activity for longer durations.

Examples of activities that primarily use the glycolysis are 200-400m sprints, a shift in hockey, and certain portions and durations of a wrestling match.

Lastly, the human body relies on the *oxidative energy system* for fuel. The oxidative energy system is primarily responsible for energy at rest and when physical activities at a more moderate intensity occur for long durations. This system requires oxygen for energy production, so it is an aerobic system. When the oxidative system is primarily being used, power output will be low but the low intensity activities can be fueled for a long duration. This system can produce ATP using either fat or carbohydrates as the substrate providing the glucose molecules (fat undergoes beta oxidation first); the selection depends on the intensity and duration of the activity. During more intense activities, the body will rely on carbohydrates since they break down faster than fats, but once the glucose is depleted, the body will start utilizing fats as the energy source. Examples activities that primarily use of the oxidative system are resting, long duration walking, and marathons.

Effects of Manipulating Training Variables

As stated previously, it is important for the strength and conditioning professional to acquire an understanding of different protocols to apply when attempting to manipulate the training adaptations of the energy systems. By acquiring this knowledge, the strength and conditioning professional will become better prepared to train the athlete's specific energy systems used in his or her sport.

During exercise, especially at higher intensities, the body uses an excessive amount of oxygen to fuel the activity. After the cessation of exercise, the body remains in a higher rate of oxygen uptake. This high oxygen uptake is termed *excess post-exercise oxygen consumption* or EPOC. The primary purpose of EPOC to restore the body to homeostasis. It is important to note that any exercise will induce EPOC, but the extent of the EPOC is highly dependent on the intensity of the activity, and secondarily on the duration over which it occurred. EPOC will be greater with higher-intensity, longer-duration exercise. Activities that last over 40 minutes have a greater EPOC than those that are of shorter durations. Many occasions will arise when the strength and conditioning professional will not be provided with enough time (over 40 minutes) to perform energy system development exercises that increase EPOC. In these occasions, different modalities can be performed to ensure the athletes are conditioning their metabolic systems.

Interval Training
Interval training uses predetermined intervals of work and rest to accommodate specific needs of the athlete, while developing the energy systems of the body. Interval training can be very useful for the strength and conditioning professional, especially when time is limited. When using interval training, the athlete can perform more work at a higher intensity than if the exercise was performed continuously. This is primarily due to the amount of rest that is interspersed with the exercise. As an example, if an athlete were to run 1600 meters all out, the time of work would be longer, and the intensity a bit lower, than if the athlete were to perform 4 sets of 400-meter sprints with 3 minutes of rest between sets. When programming energy system development protocols, it is important for the strength and conditioning professional to understand proper work-to-rest ratios for the targeted energy system. In basic terms, the work-to-rest ratio is the amount of predetermined time for the exercise to occur (work period) to the amount of predetermined time for cessation of the exercise (rest). The following are the work-to-rest ratios that are associated with specific energy system development:

- Phosphagen Energy System: 1:12–1:20
- Glycolytic Energy System: 1:3–1:5
- Oxidative Energy System: 1:1–1:3

For the energy system development program to be successful, intensity and duration must be considered. For the phosphagen system, the typical intensities at which the exercise must be performed for proper adaptation is 90-100% of maximal effort and the duration of the exercise should be 5-10 seconds. To target glycolysis, the exercise intensity should range from 75% to 90% and last 10 seconds to 2 minutes or so. For bouts that last between 1 minute and 3 minutes, the body will use a combination of the glycolytic and oxidative systems for energy. Lastly, when trying to develop the oxidative energy system, the intensities should range from 20%-80% and the duration should be 3 minutes or greater.

High Intensity Interval Training (HIIT)

High Intensity Interval Training (HIIT) is a variation of interval training that incorporates intermittent rest periods and repeated efforts of work. This technique can be very useful when time in a session is limited. Oftentimes, when incorporating HIIT, running, cycling, calisthenics, and rowing exercises are used. When used properly, HIIT can produce advantageous adaptations to metabolic, neuromuscular, and cardiopulmonary systems simultaneously. Although there are many advantages to HIIT, one must be cautious when using HIIT concurrently with other means of athletic development. HIIT can become very stressful on the body and can result in a higher incidence of injury and overtraining. Therefore, the strength and conditioning professional should incorporate HIIT activities into periods of the training cycle where stress is lower and manageable from a performance training standpoint.

Cross Training

Lastly, combination training, or cross-training, refers to training programs that combine aerobic endurance and anaerobic training. Many believe this type of training is detrimental to the anaerobic capabilities of the athlete since this training increases aerobic capacity and limits anaerobic involvement. While this may be true during periods of competition, there are many cases when combination training is suitable for the advancement of athletic performance. Early offseason is a great example of a period of the training cycle where combination training could be appropriate. During early offseason training cycles, loads are still relatively light, and the aerobic system should be developed to accommodate the recovery needs of the athlete as the progressive load increases throughout the season. Aerobic capacity can be linked with the body's ability to recover, especially in terms of potential power output; therefore, it is a training modality that can be helpful even for anaerobic athletes. When prescribing and programming aerobic endurance training, the strength and conditioning professional must consider the point of the training and competition cycle that the athlete is in as well as the demands of his or her sport. Lastly, cross-training exercises are useful for injured athletes whereby a different mode of exercise can be used to maintain fitness, so long as it does not require use of the injured body part.

Neuroendocrine Physiology

Functions of Hormones

Hormones and neuroendocrine responses can have a major impact on the adaptations that occur from training. Therefore, the strength and conditioning professional should acquire a thorough understanding of the basic concepts of the endocrine system and how different hormones respond to various training stimuli. Adaptation can occur from any stressor that is placed on the human body. This adaptation phenomenon is known as *general adaptation syndrome* or GAS. GAS describes the basic fundamental aspects of progressive overload used in athletic performance training. Anytime the body is stressed, whether from emotional, physical, or psychological stress, it will respond in a certain predictable way. Initially, the alarm response will reduce certain functions of the human body to prevent harm and focus on protecting the body from the immediate stressor. Once the alarm response occurs, an adaptation to the stress will then take place to become more suitable to handle the stress. When the stressor is exercise, such as in a hard workout, the response is termed as the *training adaptation.*

During the response phase of general adaptation syndrome, hormones will increase or decrease in the circulatory system. These hormones can have different during training and include anabolic or catabolic effects. Anabolic hormones help build molecules, cells, or tissues, such as muscle. Catabolic hormones break down molecules, cells, or tissues. Catabolic processes are especially active during overtraining or severe overreaching of the athlete. Lastly, some hormones have a more moderate effect and allow other processes to occur or not to occur; these are called permissive responses.

Hormones are chemicals that are derived from the endocrine glands of the human body. These hormones are either stored in the endocrine glands, released by the endocrine glands, or synthesized within the endocrine glands. The endocrine system of the human body consists of many glands that communicate regularly to release, store, or synthesize the hormones throughout the day. The endocrine system consists of the hypothalamus, pituitary gland, thyroid gland, parathyroid glands, heart, adrenal glands, liver, pancreas, kidneys, and the reproductive glands (ovaries in females and testes in males). Typically, the endocrine system can release hormones in two different pathways. First, a chemical signal can stimulate the endocrine gland and as a result, hormones are released. Secondly, direct neural stimulation can signal the adrenal glands to release the hormones. Once the hormones are released, they are carried within the blood and throughout the circulatory system where they can react with hormone-specific receptors, which are located on the surface.

During the training process, adaptations can occur from the release and storage of certain hormones that promote tissue building. Hormones that promote the tissue building process, especially protein synthesis, are *anabolic hormones*. Anabolic hormones include testosterone, insulin, and insulin-like growth factor. Hormones such as cortisol and glucagon are *catabolic hormones,* which have the ability to metabolize muscle proteins and degrade the tissues. During the training and adaptation process, catabolic hormones are just as important as anabolic ones because they help with the remodeling of tissue and providing immediate energy during exercise. Thyroid hormones also play an important role in the regulation of other circulating hormones during the adaptation process. Thyroid hormones are permissive hormones that can allow or block the actions of the anabolic or catabolic hormones from taking place. Without the permissive thyroid hormones, other anabolic and catabolic hormones would be consistently competing against one another. Therefore, thyroid function and thyroid health should be an important aspect of the health of any athlete.

As previously discussed, hormones are released and enter into the bloodstream where they have the ability to interact with specific receptors throughout the human body. The ability for a hormone to have one specific receptor site is known as the *lock-and-key theory.* The lock-and-key theory states that one hormone (key) can only interact with specific receptors (lock) and only those two sites can interact with each other. Although this theory is true to a certain extent, certain exceptions can occur. When a hormone has the ability to partially interact with a receptor site, and therefore block any other interaction from occurring at that site, it is termed *cross-reactivity.* Also, receptor sites can have a separate site at which other substances can affect the response of certain hormones at the target site. This separate site is termed an *allosteric binding site* and can either reduce or enhance the initial response of the hormone at the receptor site.

Once the hormone has interacted with the receptor site, the hormone will now signal the cells to respond to the hormonal stimulus. This response often affects the DNA of the specific cell or signals an increase or decrease in cellular metabolism. The response will now occur until the signal is no longer received from the hormone. When a receptor site decreases its ability to respond to a specific hormone or negates the response process altogether, it is known as downregulation of receptor function. Downregulation can greatly alter the sensitivity of the receptor, therefore changing the hormonal response of the human body.

Testosterone

For the strength and conditioning professional, anabolic and androgenic hormones are of much concern because these are the hormones responsible for the building and developing of the athlete. *Testosterone* is considered to be the primary androgen (male sex hormone) that communicates with the musculoskeletal system of the human body. When testosterone is released (originating from the testes in males and ovaries and adrenal glands from females), it enters into the circulatory system and searches for the specific receptor sites with which it can interact. Although the release of testosterone into the blood is vital, testosterone does not take effect until it reaches and interacts with the specific receptor site. The receptor sites for which testosterone can interact are located within the target tissues. Once the testosterone reaches the receptor site, it interacts with the target tissue. For muscle fibers, this causes a large increase in calcium within the fiber. This calcium increase allows stronger fiber contractions, as well as an increase in protein synthesis.

Growth Hormone

Growth hormone plays a vital role in adaptation, especially during general adaptation syndrome. Growth hormone is especially active during childhood growth and development. It is derived and released from the pituitary gland. During resistance exercises, especially those that are dependent on the Valsalva maneuver, growth hormone is released. The increase of abdominal pressure, and subsequent hypoxic environments, demonstrates that the release of growth hormone increases when exercises reach a certain intensity threshold. When this threshold is met and growth hormone is released, it enters the circulatory system, where it can begin binding to specific receptor sites. These sites are primarily found in the plasma membranes of the target cells. Growth hormone secretion tends to increase during certain hours of sleep as well.

Neuroendocrine Responses to Exercise and Training

Hormone responses can be vitally important to multiple aspects of the training program. Portions of the training cycle that focus on hypertrophy, strength, or power can have major influences on, as well as be influenced by, the hormonal profile of the athlete. Therefore, strength and conditioning professionals should acquire a thorough understanding of the endocrine responses as they relate to training, as well as specific exercises that can be incorporated to influence the desired response. During the training process, both testosterone and growth hormone concentrations can increase if the proper programming of exercise selection, volume, intensity, and rest periods are implemented.

When trying to achieve optimal hormonal response to training, the strength and conditioning professional should be aware of the exercises that elicit such responses. Using ground-based, multi-joint movements can increase blood concentrations of the anabolic hormones of the human body. Also, exercises that incorporate large muscle groups will increase blood concentrations more than exercises that utilize smaller muscle groups. Therefore, the strength and conditioning professional should incorporate exercises such as deadlifts, squats, power cleans, front squats, and Romanian deadlifts into all training programs that are geared toward stimulating the athlete's anabolic hormone action. Volume and intensity also play major roles in increasing hormonal blood concentration levels. In terms of volume, both moderate- and high-volume training sessions have been shown to increase the blood concentration levels of both testosterone and growth hormone. Volume that is adequate for such a response is multiple sets of ground-based, multi-joint exercises that use repetition ranges from 5–10. It is important to note the need for multiple sets during the training session. Single set exercises do not induce the same hormonal response as those that incorporate multiple sets, and therefore should not be used when trying to achieve maximal anabolic hormonal levels. During the individual training sessions and throughout the training process, intensities should remain high within the appropriate repetition ranges. Intensity should remain within 85–95 percent within the given repetition range. Short rest intervals have been shown to increase the hormonal response during the training process. Rest periods should range between 30 seconds and 1 minute, to elicit the desired hormonal response. Using all these factors can greatly increase the efficacy of the training program when trying to encourage positive increases in the hormonal response.

Cardiopulmonary Anatomy and Physiology

Cardiopulmonary Anatomy

During the training process, the cardiovascular system undergoes adaptations that are determined from the amount of stress that is placed on it. Therefore, the strength and conditioning professional should acquire a basic understanding of the structure and function of the cardiopulmonary system, and how it responds to the training process. Primarily, the *cardiovascular system* is responsible for the exchange of oxygen, transportation of nutrients throughout the body, and removal of waste from the cells. All of these primary responsibilities allow the cardiovascular system to maintain homeostasis of all of the body's functions.

Structures of the Heart

The heart consists of two connected pumps. The top portion of each one of these pumps is a chamber known as an *atrium*, and the lower portion of each one of these pumps is the *ventricle*. The chambers on the right side are responsible for receiving blood from the body and pumping it to the lungs for oxygenation, and the ones on the left side receive the newly oxygenated blood from the lungs and pump it out to the remainder of the body. The heart is considered a muscular organ and can undergo many of the same adaptation processes as skeletal muscles. Within the chambers are valves that allow, or block, the blood flow during ventricle contraction. Contraction of the heart is known as *systole*, and relaxation of the ventricle is known as *diastole*. During systole, the bicuspid valve and tricuspid valve prevent the blood from reentering the atria from the ventricles. The tricuspid valve and bicuspid valve, collectively, are known as the *atrioventricular valves*. During diastolic relaxation, the aortic valve and pulmonary valve prevent the backflow of blood from the arteries into the ventricles. The aortic valve and pulmonary valve, collectively, are known as the *semilunar valves*.

An electrical impulse, during contraction and relaxation of the heart, enables the conduction system to efficiently pump blood throughout the body. This conduction system comprises many structures that ensure the rhythm is constant even if the rate of the heart beat increases with exertion. The *sinoatrial node (SA node)* is the starting place of the electrical impulse and is known as the biological pacemaker of the conduction system. The impulse is then sent, via the internodal pathways, from the SA node to the *atrioventricular node (AV node)*. The AV node slightly delays the impulse before sending it further to the *atrioventricular bundle (AV bundle)*. The AV bundle is the location where the impulse is prepared to be conducted to the ventricles of the heart. Once prepared, the impulse can be sent to the left and right bundle branches of the heart. Finally, the impulse divides and is conducted into the Purkinje fibers, which allows both ventricles to receive the impulse.

The conduction system, as well as the electrical impulse, can be observed through a graph known as an electrocardiogram (ECG). The graph that is displayed during an electrocardiogram comprises a P-wave, a QRS complex (Q-wave, R-wave, S-wave), and a T-wave. Throughout contraction and relaxation, the heart undergoes depolarization and repolarization. Depolarization occurs when the negative potential inside the membrane becomes positive and the outside potential becomes positive. Repolarization occurs when the ventricles restore homeostasis throughout conduction. The P-wave and QRS complex can be observed during the ECG and represent the depolarization phase of the heart. Furthermore, the T-wave that occurs following the P-wave and QRS complex represents the repolarization phase of contraction.

The Structure of the Heart and the Path of Blood Flow

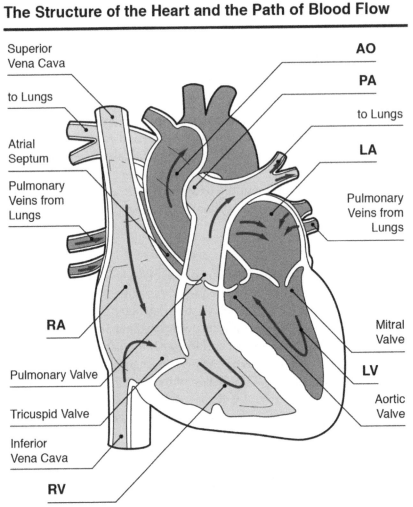

Vascular System

The primary role of the cardiovascular system is to transport nutrients to the cells of the body and return waste to the lungs where it can be removed. Blood is the main vehicle in which the nutrients and waste products are transported. Oxygen within the blood is transported via an iron-protein molecule called *hemoglobin* that is located within the red blood cells. The transportation of blood throughout the human body is accomplished by two primary systems: the arterial system and the venous system. The *arterial system* transports blood away from the heart and to the rest of the body. The *venous system* transports blood from the body to the heart. These systems are interconnected and work together, efficiently, to accomplish the roles of the cardiovascular system.

The arterial system begins with arteries. Arteries are large and strong vasculature because they need to withstand the velocity and force with which the heart pumps. Further from the heart, large arteries become smaller *arterioles*, which act as a control center by allowing or preventing the volume of blood entering into the capillaries. The nutrient-dense blood then reaches the *capillaries*, which are thin, permeable vessels that allow gas exchange between the cells and tissues of the body. The permeability of the capillaries allows tissue to receive many substances such as hormones, fluid, nutrients, electrolytes, and oxygen.

Once these substances are used by the tissues, the blood then begins to pool back into the capillaries where it will begin transport back to the heart and lungs via the venous system. The venous system comprises transport vessels that have thin walls, as the pressure of the blood returning to the heart is low. This system starts with *venules*, which collect the blood in the capillaries and begin transporting it to the larger vessels of the venous system, which are known as *veins*. Blood merges in the veins and returns to the right atrium of the heart so that it can enter pulmonary circulation so it can be rid of the waste products (primarily carbon dioxide) and re-oxygenate to begin the process again.

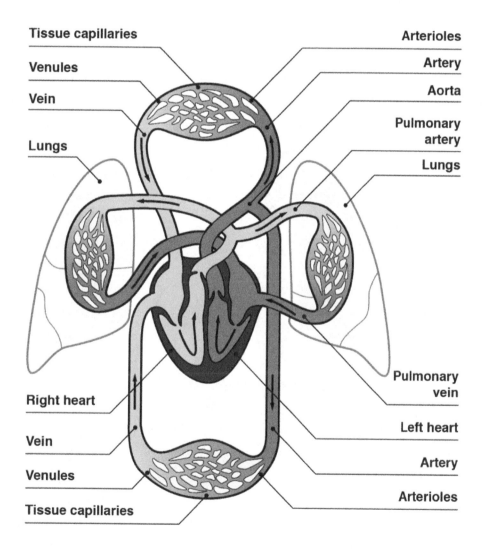

Respiratory System
The of gaseous exchange between the air and the body is the primary role of the *respiratory system*. This system allows the cells and tissues of the body to receive oxygen and expel carbon dioxide through daily activities. The inhalation of air begins in the nose. The naval cavities receive the air, where it is then

humidified, purified, and warmed. The air then moves to the first-generation passage known as the *trachea*. The trachea splits into the left and right main bronchi. The left and right main bronchi bring the inspired air into the lungs, where it undergoes separation into advanced generations known as *bronchioles*. Once the inspired air is transported throughout the bronchioles, it then reaches the *alveoli*. The alveoli are the last generation and the location where the gases are exchanged during respiration. Once the oxygen reaches the alveoli, it diffuses into the pulmonary blood. Diffusion occurs when molecules move from one location of higher concentration to an area of lower concentration. During respiration, this occurs when oxygen diffuses from the alveoli to the pulmonary blood, or when carbon dioxide diffuses from the pulmonary blood to the alveoli. During respiration, the diffusion process occurs when gases are transitioned from areas of high concentrations to areas of low concentrations. Therefore, the exchange rate is highly dependent on the concentrations of gases within the alveoli and capillaries.

Respiratory System

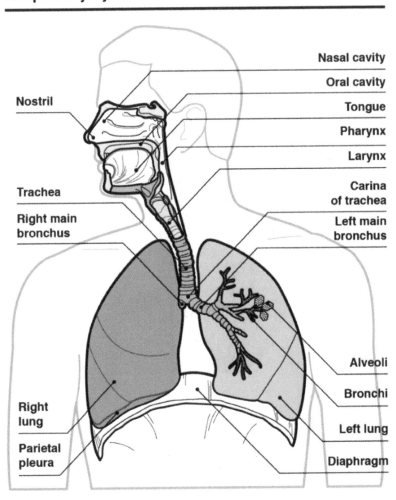

During respiration, the lungs expand and retract to control the volume of air within the system. The expansion and retraction are controlled by two different mechanisms: the upward and downward movement of the diaphragm and the depression and elevation of the ribs. During nonstrenuous activities, as well as at rest, the lungs are primarily controlled by the movement of the diaphragm. During strenuous activities, respiration becomes deeper and faster and is controlled by the diaphragm, assisted by the abdominal muscles and the elevation of the rib cage. By elevating the rib cage, the sternum is allowed to move forward and away from the spine, allowing more expansion of the lungs.

Cardiopulmonary Responses to Exercise and Training

Many adaptations can occur within the cardiopulmonary system during training. Adaptations in heart rate, oxygen uptake, cardiac output, stroke volume, blood pressure, and vasodilation have all been observed as a benefit of training. Therefore, it is important for the strength and conditioning professional to understand the different training modalities and their role in causing adaptations of the cardiopulmonary system.

Slightly prior to activity, and during the onset of exercise, the body's heart rate will increase due to the anticipatory response of the central nervous system. This increase will continue with the continuation of exercise but will be dependent on the intensity and workload of the muscles being utilized throughout the acute training bout. The maximal heart rate achieved through training is dependent on the current fitness level of the athlete, as well as his or her age. As the body adapts and achieves higher fitness levels, a slight increase in maximal heart rate can be reached. Maximal heart rate decreases as age increases.

Oxygen uptake relates to the amount of oxygen that can be used by the tissues of the human body. During training, oxygen uptake increases as the muscle tissues perform at higher rates. The amount of oxygen used is dependent on the size of the musculature being used, the mitochondrial density in the muscle fibers, and the intensity at which the exercise is being performed. Aerobic training tends to increase oxygen uptake more than anaerobic training. Maximal oxygen uptake is the total amount of oxygen the cells can utilize for the entire human body and is a great indicator of an athlete's aerobic conditioning. Higher maximal oxygen uptake correlates to an increase in overall conditioning levels, as well as an increased ability to recover from intense training sessions.

During training sessions, especially when utilizing aerobic exercise modalities, an increase is observed in both cardiac output and stroke volume. As muscles are performing work, the need for oxygenated blood increases. Therefore, cardiac output will rise proportionally to the intensity and workload of the exercise. *Cardiac output* is the total volume of blood that is pumped by the heart, and *stroke volume* is the volume of blood ejected for each beat. Both cardiac output and stroke volume increase as exercise occurs, but cardiac output increases rapidly, begins to taper off, and then reaches a plateau. Stroke volume increases from the onset of exercise, and consistently increases until oxygen utilization is approximately 45 percent, before beginning to plateau. Overtime, stroke volume can increase in response to regular training, allowing for heart rates at submaximal levels to decrease.

Local circulation of blood and blood pressure both respond to exercise and training. During bouts of exercise, the need for oxygenated blood increases. Therefore, the blood vessels undergo dilatation to allow a greater volume to be circulated to the working tissues. This dilation process of the blood vessels is termed *vasodilation*. During rest, blood flow to skeletal muscle is approximately 15–20 percent of total blood volume. As physical demands increase, the amount of blood distributed to the muscles also increases and can reach upward of 90 percent of total cardiac output when intensities are high enough. Furthermore, as the need for oxygenated blood increases, an increase in systolic blood pressure can be observed. Normal systolic blood pressure is approximately 110 mmHg, though it is considered healthy as long as it is 120 mmHg or below. Diastolic blood pressure should be at or below 80 mmHg to be considered healthy. Although hypertension used to be considered defined as a blood pressure of greater than or equal to 140/90 mmHg, it is now defined as ≥130/80 mm Hg. Like many other variables that rise with physical exertion, systolic blood pressure increases as more blood is forcefully ejected from the heart to fill the need for more oxygenated blood by the working tissues. During exercise, changes can usually only be observed in systolic blood pressure, as contraction ejects blood away from the heart. Therefore, diastolic blood pressure is generally nonresponsive during training.

Physiological Adaptations to Exercise and Training

Adaptations to Metabolic Conditioning

Metabolic adaptations can result from proper exercise training. Therefore, strength and conditioning professionals must acquire an understanding of the adaptations that can result from specific conditioning activities to adequately accommodate the needs of athletes for their particular events. *Metabolic conditioning* refers to activities that increase the body's ability to create, utilize, replenish, and expend energy during and after exercise. In accordance to general adaptation syndrome, the body responds and adequately adapts to the stress that is placed upon it. Therefore, it is important to prescribe conditioning activities that target the energy system of the athlete's sport.

Through the use of metabolic conditioning activities, the body undergoes many adaptations to accommodate the stress and increase its physical readiness for the event of another similar training stimulus. The ability to recover quickly from a bout of exercise is one of the first adaptations that the body undergoes. When given ample amount of time to rest, the body will adapt by increasing its ability to withstand repeated bouts and increased intensity. Therefore, an increase in work capacity is usually the first sign of adaptation to metabolic conditioning activities. As previously described, the endocrine system responds accordingly to the physical stress of the training program. Furthermore, metabolic conditioning has been shown to cause adaptations in the hormonal response of the body. The activity of hormones that are responsible in metabolism regulation increase when metabolic conditioning activities are properly programed into the training regimen. In addition, cortisol increases more in untrained athletes than in trained athletes during metabolic conditioning exercises. Therefore, it can be concluded that an adaptation to metabolic conditioning is enhanced cortisol resistance in trained individuals.

Optimal energy utilization is another adaptation to metabolic conditioning. As the body responds to the training stimulus, the energy-generating pathways coincide with the energy demands of the activity become more efficient or even more plentiful. For example, mitochondrial density can increase in type 1 muscle fibers with aerobic training. This allows the muscles to generate more energy via oxidative metabolism. As adaptations occur, the reliance on carbohydrates for energy decreases while the body becomes more efficient at utilizing fat. Each of these adaptations is a positive response in the body's generation and use of ATP. Therefore, metabolic conditioning, when applied appropriately for the specific sport, can be an important training advantage when physically preparing an athlete for a specific sporting event.

Causes, Signs, Symptoms, and Effects of Overtraining and Detraining

Consistently applying stress and allowing adaptation is one of the major roles of a strength and conditioning professional. While this is essential, it is also important to understand and recognize the symptoms of overtaxing the body, or of not giving the body enough time to adapt to the stress before applying the stress again.

Overtraining
Pushing the body through training can be positive, as this is what ultimately leads to physiological adaptations. However, training too intensely can also have detrimental effects. Common terms for overuse

are functional overreaching and nonfunctional overreaching. Both are forms of overuse, but have very different effects on the body in terms of long-term progress. *Functional overreaching* refers to increasing stress on the body until no further stress can be placed on it without a period of recovery. This is usually planned in a period of loading stress on the athlete, followed by a period of rest, commonly referred to as a *de-load period*. When the load reaches a peak and is not followed by a period of de-load, stress becomes too high and detrimental consequences can occur to the athlete. If the detrimental consequences occur over an extended period of time without a proper recovery period, the athlete may become overtrained. *Overtraining* refers to maladaptation within the training process over a significant time period; recovery from this problem can take a significant amount of time (as long as 6 to 8 months). There are two distinct categories of overtraining: sympathetic overtraining syndrome and parasympathetic overtraining syndrome. During *sympathetic overtraining syndrome*, sympathetic activity is increased during periods of rest, whereas during *parasympathetic overtraining syndrome*, parasympathetic activity is increased during periods of rest. An athlete can usually recover more quickly from sympathetic overtraining syndrome and is it oftentimes observed as a precursor to parasympathetic overtraining syndrome. For the strength and conditioning professional, it is important to be able to identify the signs and symptoms of overtraining. Early identification can result in adjusting the training program to adequately provide enough recovery to accommodate and restore the biological functions associated with overtraining syndrome. The following are signs and symptoms of overtraining:

- Emotional disturbances
- Decrease in sleep performance
- Increase in illness and immune suppression
- Hormonal imbalances
- Anemia
- High rate of perceived exertion within training
- Loss of appetite
- Common injuries (lack of durability)
- Allergies
- Onset of asthma or asthma related symptoms
- Persistent fatigue that cannot be attributed to any other stimulus
- Social disturbances from family, relationships, team, or work
- Endocrine disorders

Detraining
The cessation of training and the negative effects on the physical attributes attained from the previously performed training program is termed as *detraining*. When the physical stress is removed, the body responds by regressing toward an untrained status. The result of this regression is partial or complete loss of the positive adaptations that resulted from a proper and specific training program. For strength and conditioning professionals working in high school and collegiate settings, detraining can occur during academic break periods. Therefore, it is important for the strength and conditioning professional to understand the maximal amount of time of inactivity before fitness gains begin to decline. The following list shows the maximum duration (in days) that residual effects for certain physical attributes will remain despite stopping training:

- Aerobic endurance: 30 +/- 5
- Maximal strength: 30 +/- 5
- Anaerobic endurance: 18 +/- 4
- Strength endurance: 15 +/- 5
- Maximal speed: 5 +/- 5

Given the previous information, when periods of inactivity are longer than those associated with the residual effects, the strength and conditioning professional must be cognizant that the athlete has likely lost fitness and the program will need to be adjusted accordingly.

Anatomical, Physiological, and Biomechanical Differences of Athletes

When designing training programs, it is important to develop the training protocols around the needs of the athlete. Therefore, it is important to understand the anatomical, physiological, and biomechanical differences among athletes of different biological ages, sexes, and training ages while still being conducive to their sporting activities. Although many athletes have similarities, in both trainability and sport, certain differences must be considered to ensure a safe and effective training program.

Biological Age

For the strength and conditioning professional, age can play a major role in the administration of training techniques as well as the selection of specific exercises. It is important to understand that children and adolescents do not respond in the same manner to certain training protocols as do adults. Furthermore, older adults, such as the geriatric population, require modifications to certain training protocols to ensure the training regimen is safe and effective. Therefore, biological age (the functional age of the body and its structures and systems), as well as chronological age, should be considered when designing programs for children, adolescents, and the geriatric population.

Children and adolescents are consistently increasing their participation in athletic physical development. Therefore, the strength and conditioning professional must understand the differences between training the general athletic population and that of the children and adolescent population. To start, the youth population is still developing their bone structure and function. Growth plates within bones are not fully developed and may become damaged if exercise selection, technical progressions, or load progressions are too aggressive or inappropriate. Furthermore, the hormonal response to exercise is not the same as that of the general adult athletic population. In prepubescent children, circulating hormones such as testosterone, growth hormone, and insulin-like growth factor are limited. Therefore, many of the strength gains witnessed during training programs are that of increased hypertrophy of the musculature and neural factors. To ensure that appropriate training programs are administered to the youth population, the strength and conditioning professional should follow certain guidelines:

1. Make sure the youth athlete understands the benefits and risks associated with the training program.

2. Closely monitor youth athletes at all times when performing each exercise, and never leave them alone during the training session.

3. Require youth athletes to perform an appropriate and thorough warmup prior to any resistance training.

4. Closely monitor youth athletes' exercise stress response.

5. Assign appropriate levels of exercise (1-3 sets of 6-15 repetitions for most youth).

6. Make subtle increases in resistance to prevent overexertion.

7. Progress technical, multi-joint movements based on the technical proficiency of the athlete.

8. Follow proper periodization throughout each exercise.

Just as in youth participation in resistance training, older athletes are furthering their athletic endeavors in later stages in life. It is not uncommon to see athletes over the age of 65 compete in weightlifting competitions and marathons, as well as other sporting events. Therefore, the strength and conditioning professional must understand the anatomical, physiological, and biomechanical implications that are associated with the geriatric athletic community.

Advancing age of the participants can be associated with muscle mass loss, which is known as *sarcopenia*. The muscle mass loss, as well as the rate at which it is lost, can be largely due to inactivity of the athlete. Therefore, it is important for older adults to maintain physical activity as they age. When muscle mass is lost, muscular strength and power of the athlete also decline. Cross-sectional areas of muscles begin to decrease after the age of 30 or so and will continue to decline if the athlete does not partake in an appropriate resistance training program. Furthermore, neuromotor function also begins to decline with age and can be related to many of the falls, dislocations, and skeletal fractures that become common in older adults. With these factors in mind, the strength and conditioning professional should follow certain guidelines when programming a training regimen for older athletes:

1. Prior to activity, older adult athletes should undergo a thorough pre-activity screening to account for any potential known or previously undiagnosed medical issues.

2. Warmups should be thorough and comprehensive to account for lower blood circulation.

3. Dynamic stretching should precede workouts and static stretching should follow to aid flexibility.

4. Resistance of exercises should not be overtaxing, and appropriate periodization protocols should be used.

5. The Valsalva maneuver should be used sparingly to prevent an increase in blood pressure.

6. Recovery from individual training sessions should be closely monitored to allow the body to fully recover prior to partaking in another training session that uses the same musculature or physiological systems.

7. Only qualified strength and conditioning professionals should program, teach, and monitor the training of older adults.

Sex

Sex-related differences between males and females need to be considered when designing safe and effective training protocols for athletes. Therefore, it is important that the strength and conditioning professional acquire a basic understanding in commonalties and differences between males and females prior to designing training regimens for athletes.

Prepubescent male and female bodies have fewer differences in physical characteristics than adult males and females. As the athletes undergo puberty, the hormonal response is very different between the two sexes and subsequent development diverges significantly. Males experience an increase in testosterone during this period. This increase in testosterone is responsible for increases in muscle mass and bone formation. During puberty, females experience increases in estrogen, which increases their body fat and begins the development of secondary sex characteristics like breast tissue growth. After going through puberty, males typically have more muscle mass, weigh more in total weight, and have higher bone density compared to their prepubescent bodies as well as to the typical post-puberty female body. Females tend to be lighter in body weight, have less muscle mass, higher body fat percentages, and lower bone density than that of males. Their pelvises also tend to be wider. It is important to note that although males generally have more muscle mass than females, the quality of muscle tends to be the same, on average. Furthermore, although quality of muscle mass tends to be equal, males display more ability for strength and power due to the quantity of muscle mass.

Although males and females do have sex-related differences, they both tend to respond similarly to resistance training protocols. Although the initial strength and power of females is less than that of males, both sexes can progress in strength and power at similar rates. Taking this into account, the strength and conditioning professional can program around the individual needs of the athlete instead of the specific sex of the athlete.

Training Status and Sport Specificity

When designing training programs for athletic physical development, the strength and conditioning professional must understand the current training status of the athlete, as well as the physical demands and characteristics of the sport. Although sport specificity is important, many exercises can be utilized across lots of different sports. As an example, the need for strong hip extensors is important across all sports that require running (as well as many others); therefore, similar exercises can be used in the attainment of this attribute.

Understanding the current training status can be imperative to a safe and effective training program. Therefore, the strength and conditioning professional should acquire knowledge from participants about their previously performed training regimen, as well as their readiness to train. After this knowledge is acquired, athletes should undergo a basic prescreening prior to partaking in any exercise training protocol. Furthermore, new exercises should be thoroughly taught before external resistance is added to the movement. Neglecting to instruct proper movement mechanics and quickly adding resistance can be detrimental to the physical development of the athlete. Once movements are taught, the athlete should then perform an appropriate progression, ensuring that proper technique is maintained throughout the maneuvers.

As previously stated, many exercises can be helpful for a range of different sports. The need for total body strength and power is a commonality across many sports. Therefore, the strength and conditioning professional must design programs that address general fitness as well as the specific needs of the athlete. Two areas that must be addressed, when designing programs for specific sports, are the prevention of common injuries that can occur during the sporting activity and the specific energy demands that are used within the sport. Therefore, special attention in the training program should be placed on injury prevention. Furthermore, conditioning activities should resemble the energy demands of the sporting activity. When designing conditioning activities, the strength and conditioning professional must understand the primary and secondary energy systems that are used within the sport and apply specific activities that coincide with these systems. By designing training programs that are specific to the athlete's needs, applying injury prevention protocols based around the individual's sport, and conditioning the metabolic pathways necessary for the sporting activity, the strength and conditioning professional can ensure that the training program is appropriate for the attainment of enhanced performance ability for the athlete.

Psychological Techniques Used to Enhance Training and Performance

Athletic success can be attributed to four main components: tactical, technical, physical, and psychological. If, at any time, one of these four main components is lacking, the athlete may not perform to their potential. Therefore, with any athletic development program that encompasses the entire athletic needs of the athlete, each of these components must be addressed. One of the most important components is psychological, although it is often overlooked by strength and conditioning professionals if they do not understand all that entails the psychological wellbeing of the athlete. Therefore, it is imperative that strength and conditioning professionals acquire a thorough understanding of strategies and techniques used for optimal sport psychology.

Motivational Techniques

The intensity of mental effort and the focus of that effort is known as *motivation*. Motivation for competition and training, as well as a desire to be successful, can have major implications for the outcome of an athletic career. When observing motivation, successful athletes demonstrate both intrinsic and extrinsic motivation. *Intrinsic motivation* relates to the internal desire to be successful, love for the sport, and the internal reward the athlete perceives for his or her participation. *Extrinsic motivation* relates to the desire for external rewards from successful outcomes of training and competition. Examples of extrinsic motivation include social acceptance, trophies, awards, induction into a hall of fame, praise from fans or friends, praise from coaches, and threat of punishment for an unwanted outcome in training and competition. It is important to note that athletes are usually not solely motivated by intrinsic or extrinsic factors, but rather a combination of both. Therefore, it is important for the strength and conditioning professional to assess the motivation of each athlete and provide support that aligns with the individualized motivation factors of the athlete.

Achievement motivation is a specialized form of motivation that relates to the athlete's desire for skill mastery, overcoming obstacles, achieving excellence, and engaging in competition. Attaining this type of motivation can be very beneficial to athletes, as it will increase their desire for competition and to achieve greater success. Furthermore, achievement motivation is broken down into two subcategories: *motive to achieve success (MAS)* and *motive to avoid failure (MAF)*. MAS is an athletic motive where the athlete desires to experience pride and self-worth in their personal accomplishments, therefore embracing ever-increasing personal challenges and consistently evaluating themselves by the outcome of these challenges. MAF is a motive for the athlete to protect their ego, self-worth, and self-esteem. It is important to note that MAF is not a motive to avoid failure necessarily, but instead to avoid the perception of shame from teammates, coaches, fans, and family. Athletes with a high MAS seem to perform well in situations that are challenging and when the known outcome is uncertain. Athletes with a high MAF often seek out competitions that are easy and unchallenging to them personally. As competitors are observed in elite levels of competition, athletes that are MAS-dominant are more likely to achieve success because they seem to thrive in challenging situations and competitions.

Reinforcement Techniques

Throughout the training cycle, as well as athletic competitions, the strength and conditioning coach may benefit from the use of reinforcement techniques to induce the desired outcomes. An *operant* is a specific outcome that is targeted through stimulus conditioning. An operant can be positive or negative, depending on the type of behavior. It is important to note that an operant is not initially the result of a specific stimulus, but rather a behavior that occurs spontaneously. It is through the different reinforcing or deterring techniques (or consequences from the operant) that the operant becomes the targeted outcome of a stimulus. Four different reinforcement techniques can be used to reinforce the operant and increase the probability of its occurrence. These techniques are positive reinforcement, negative reinforcement, positive punishment, and negative punishment.

To begin, *positive reinforcement* is the act of increasing the probability of the operant. Once the operant is observed, the strength and conditioning professional gives praise, an award, a prize, or any other positive gift for the occurrence of the operant. *Negative reinforcement* is very similar to positive reinforcement, but instead of giving the athlete a positive gift, the strength and conditioning professional removes a certain element that the athlete views negatively. An example of this is if athletes complete all main movements within a session with perfect form, then they wouldn't have to perform the sled drills at the end of the session. By removing the negative element, the operant could increase in probability of occurrence.

Besides positive reinforcement and negative reinforcement, positive punishment and negative punishment are also considered reinforcement techniques that are utilized within the strength and conditioning profession. By administering punishment reinforcement techniques, the strength and conditioning professional attempts to decrease the occurrence of a given operant. The operant being displayed is often considered negative, therefore the decrease in occurrence would increase the success of the athlete. *Positive punishment* relates to administering undesirable tasks, objects, or events that would likely decrease the occurrence of the negative operant. As an example, the strength and conditioning coach would require sprints for every missed repetition throughout the training session. Therefore, the reprimanding sprints would likely motivate the athletes to try and decrease the occurrence of missed repetitions. Contrary to positive punishment is negative punishment. *Negative punishment* is the removal of a valued object to decrease the likelihood of displaying the negative operant. This could be in the form of reducing playing time or revoking privileges within the weight room.

Strength and conditioning professionals will likely utilize all reinforcement techniques to increase the occurrence of desired behavior. It is important to understand that reinforcement techniques often have more positive outcomes than punishment techniques. Therefore, the strength and conditioning professional should use reprimanding punishment sparingly when administering reinforcement techniques with athletes.

Imagery Techniques
Another technique used to increase motivation and success within athletics is that of mental imagery. *Mental imagery* is the act of recreating successful athletic events within the mind of the athlete. This recreation entails every sensory aspect of the event: What does the athlete hear? What does the athlete see? How does the successful moment feel? What are the distinct smells of the successful event? By recreating a successful athletic endeavor, the athlete will increase the desire to actually experience such events within his or her athletic career. The mental image is not limited to competition and can include proper practice, or rehearsal, in preparation for the event. It can also include a mental rehearsal of a proper pregame ritual and how the proper pregame ritual will increase the likelihood of a successful athletic endeavor. By using mental imagery as a motivation technique, the strength and conditioning professional can increase the likelihood of positive outcomes within athletic events, and therefore increase performance during the preparation for the events.

Methods that Enhance Motor Learning and Skill Acquisition

Within the realm of sports psychology, motor learning and skill acquisition become vitally important, especially when teaching new movement patterns to novice athletes. Therefore, the strength and conditioning professional must attain knowledge in different learning techniques and methods to enhance these traits within athletics.

Instruction

The means by which the strength and conditioning professional instructs the athletes can greatly enhance the skill acquisition of the athlete. Furthermore, the delivery of the instructions can dictate the pace at which the athletes learn new movement patterns, as well as specific training exercises. Throughout learning periods, the strength and conditioning professional must be cognizant of the amount of detail given to the athlete at a certain time. Information overload can halt learning ability and slow progress within learning periods. When determining the instructional style of the motor learning and skill acquisition period, the strength and conditioning professional should assess the learning style of the athlete and design the teaching style around the individual athlete. Generally, instructional styles can be categorized in the following ways: explicit instruction, guided discovery, and discovery.

Explicit instruction relates to implementing specific tasks during the movement or exercise. The strength and conditioning professional instructs the athlete on each aspect of the movement and the athlete is then expected to demonstrate the movement. Although this instructional technique works well with some athletes, too much information could negatively alter the learning ability during the instruction period. *Guided discovery* is very similar to explicit instruction but limits the amount of information given to the athlete. Because one of the main drawbacks of explicit instruction is information overload, guided discovery gives the athlete the main information of the movement but allows athletes to learn certain aspects as they are performing the movement. The information given during guided often relates to preventing injury during the movement, but the remaining information is left for the athlete to discover. This technique is frequently used by the strength and conditioning professional with great success. *Discovery* instructs the athlete on the goal of the task, but little information is given beyond the goal. This instructional style should be used sparingly as many faults could occur, especially during the learning periods of new exercises. It is important to note that each of these styles could be used with a single athlete during the learning period. Furthermore, it is important to assess the learning style of the athlete and match that to the instruction style for optimal learning experiences.

Feedback

Throughout training, especially in learning periods, feedback can have a major impact in eliciting desired movement patterns within specific exercises. *Feedback* relates to providing the athlete with information about the movements patterns of each repetition. The information provided within the feedback can then be used to correct any errors that occurred during the movement of the exercises. Feedback can be received in two different ways: intrinsic feedback and augmented feedback. *Intrinsic feedback* occurs within the athlete's body via the proprioceptors within the musculature and tendons. Intrinsic feedback is provided by the athlete, to the athlete, and does not include information provided by the strength and conditioning professional. When information is provided by the strength and conditioning professional, it is known as *augmented feedback*. Augmented feedback is given to the athlete from the strength and conditioning professional to either reinforce adequate movement patterns or to correct faulty movement mechanics.

Augmented feedback is divided into two subcategories: knowledge of results and knowledge of performance. *Knowledge of results* allows feedback on performance based on the results of the movement. Oftentimes, knowledge of results is used in settings where the athlete is timed for a specific task. When using knowledge of results as feedback, the strength and conditioning coach should either give normative times for the exercise or give the athlete a goal to achieve. Using the 40-yard dash as an example, prior to starting the task, the coach would give the athlete a normative time based around the sport or position of the athlete. After the 40-yard dash is run, the athlete would then be told what his or her time was and how it relates to the normative time of the run. By administering knowledge of results as feedback, athlete can motivate themselves to achieve greater skill learning throughout the training process. Exercises that are not timed or when athletes receive augmented feedback about the specific movement pattern is known as *knowledge of performance*. Knowledge of performance can be delivered directly from the coach, from video analysis of the movement, or from specialized equipment such as a tendo-unit or force plate. As in many instances, overlap of augmented feedback categories often exist and the strength and conditioning professional must assess the individual and perform feedback techniques that are best suited to the athlete.

Whole Versus Part Practice

Oftentimes, complex movement patterns are incorporated within the training cycle of athletes. Therefore, the strength and conditioning professional must determine the best approach in teaching these complex movement skills to athletes. Whole practice and part practice should be considered when approaching the skill acquisition of complex movements and determining the best approach in teaching the movement mechanics of the exercises.

Whole practice tends to teach movements in their entirety. When whole practice teaching occurs, the movements are taught in one fluid movement, as the individual parts of the movement are too interrelated to separate. Whole practice instruction is best suited for movements that require use of related musculature and joints. Exercises such as squats, bench presses, and lunges are good examples of movements that are best suited for whole practice instruction. When complex movements that require use of multiple muscle groups and joints are used, *part practice* instruction may be more conducive to the skill acquisition of the movement. Exercises such as Olympic cleans and snatches often use part practice instruction for acquisition of proper technique. In part practice instruction, each segment of the movement can be broken down into subcomponents to ensure each segment is taught prior to moving into the movement as a whole. Understanding each component of each exercise incorporated in training is important when determining the use of whole practice or part practice. Therefore, the strength and conditioning professional must assess the individual, as well as the team, when determining the best plan of action for skill acquisition within the training cycle.

Attention Control and Decision Making

Focus

Throughout the training cycle, focus and attention can shift from vital aspects of performance to those of less importance. Therefore, the strength and conditioning professional should have a basic understanding of attention control and how the athlete's attention can affect his or her decision-making skills. *Attention* is the operation of processing environmental, external clues, and internal cues that come to awareness through conscious thought. Throughout training and competition, many of these cues move in and out of the athlete's awareness. It is imperative that the athlete keep their conscious thought on task-relevant stimuli. The ability to do this is known as *selective attention* or *level of focus*. When the attention is shifted to task-irrelevant stimuli, achieving the desired outcome of the task becomes far more difficult. Therefore, the strength and conditioning professional should incorporate cues and activities that strengthen cue-recognition skills of the athlete as well as ways to appropriately respond to the detected cues.

Arousal Management

Arousal relates to the athlete's psychological and physiological state at any given time. For most athletes, *high arousal* is often perceived as an increase in mental activation, positive thinking, and the ability to control decision-making tasks. On the contrary, a *low arousal* state can be associated with minimal mental activation, boredom, wandering thoughts, and a low physiological output. Throughout training, it is important to understand the arousal state of the athlete and determine the training necessary to elicit positive performance gains.

Optimal arousal states can differ greatly between athletes. Therefore, the strength and conditioning professional should administer training modalities and coaching styles based upon the optimal arousal level of the individual athlete. Although higher arousal levels are associated with higher performance outcomes, heightened arousal states are finite and can become detrimental if the arousal level becomes too high. The inverted-U theory can accurately describe this phenomenon. The *inverted-U theory* states that arousal levels increase performance up to an optimal level, but further increases in arousal are associated with reduced performance. Below is an illustration of the inverted-U theory associated with different types of athletes.

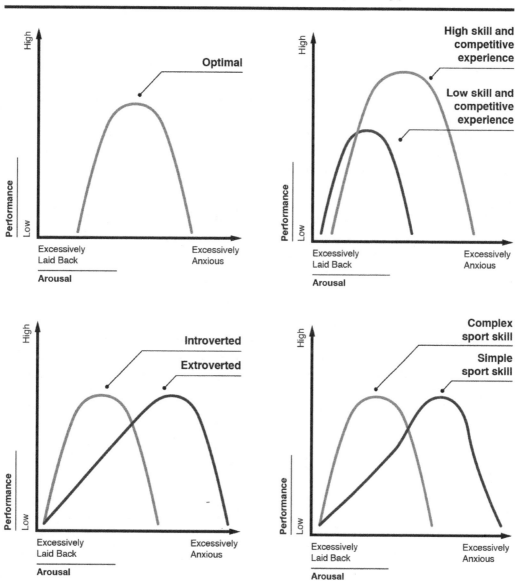

The Inverted-U Theory Associated with Different Types of Athletes

Confidence and Positive Self-Talk

Confidence

Confidence and positive self-talk can attribute to the success of the athlete. With all other attributes being the same, the athlete with the most confidence will become more successful than less confident athletes. Knowing this, the strength and conditioning professional should incorporate strategies and modalities that increase the confidence of their athletes throughout the training process. *Self-confidence* is defined as an internal belief that an athlete possesses the attributes to successfully perform a desired behavior. Furthermore, when self-confidence coincides with a specific situation or environment, it is defined as *self-efficacy*. An athlete that possess both self-confidence and self-efficacy believes he or she will be successful regardless of the situation. This confidence and efficacy holds true even when failure occurs or if a loss is sustained. When observing an athlete's confidence and efficacy levels, common occurrences can be seen:

- Remembering accomplishments in previous performances
- Watching success of others and modeling their performance
- Engaging in positive self-talk
- Using successful imagery and visualization
- Evidencing positive emotional state
- Demonstrating a favorable physiological state

For the strength and conditioning professional, it is important to review the previous confidence-boosting strategies for a given athlete and try to develop and enhance these during future training. Using exercises and movements that ensure success can be one strategy when trying to develop self-confidence in athletes. Having the athlete first perform movements that require less technical skill, and then progress to more difficult tasks can greatly enhance the confidence level of the athlete.

Positive Self-Talk

Throughout daily activities, and especially during training and competition, an internal dialogue of thoughts is continuously occurring within the athlete's mind. This internal dialogue is known as *self-talk* and can have a major impact on the athlete's mood and psyche. To ensure self-talk enables positive outcomes in both training and competition, the strength and conditioning professional should ensure that the self-talk remains positive. If at any time the self-talk becomes negative, detrimental outcomes often occur within training and competition. Therefore, athletes should develop an internal dialogue of positive phrases that accommodate successful performances. Examples of phrases that could be used are, "I'm ready," "I am prepared," "I can do this," or simply, "Come on." Each phrase may elicit a different response in individual athletes, and the response may be negative, if based on past experiences. Therefore, the strength and conditioning professional and the athlete, together, should develop these phrases to ensure they elicit the desired response.

Practice Questions

1. What is the term used for stress that is applied to the body until performance begins to decline before a period of rest?
   - a. Functional overreaching
   - b. Non-functional overreaching
   - c. Overtraining
   - d. Detraining

2. Implementation of specific tasks during athletic movements or specific exercises is known as which of the following?
   - a. Discovery
   - b. Explicit instruction
   - c. Specific instruction
   - d. Guided Discovery

3. Which of the following muscle actions is occurring in the pectoralis major as the weight is lowered to the chest in a barbell bench press exercise?
   - a. Isometric muscle action
   - b. Isokenetic muscle action
   - c. Eccentric muscle action
   - d. Concentric muscle action

4. Which of the following is NOT a component of an electrocardiogram?
   - a. P-wave
   - b. T-wave
   - c. QRS complex
   - d. U-wave

5. Which of the following is NOT a mechanism for expansion and retraction of the lungs?
   - a. Upward movement of the diaphragm
   - b. Downward movement of the diaphragm
   - c. Elevation of the ribs
   - d. Relaxation of the abdominal muscles

6. The operation of processing environmental, external, and internal cues that come to one's awareness is known as which of the following?
   - a. Conscious thinking
   - b. Attention
   - c. Subconscious thinking
   - d. Mindful engrossment

7. Which of the following encompasses the components of the axial skeleton?
   - a. Bones of the hips, knees, and ankles
   - b. Bones of the pelvic girdle, shoulder girdle, arms, and legs
   - c. Bones of the ribs, sternum, vertebral column, and skull
   - d. Bones of the hands, feet, wrists, and ankles

8. During training, children and adolescents often see an increase in performance primarily due to which of the following adaptations?
    a. Neural adaptations
    b. Muscular strength adaptations
    c. Reactive adaptations
    d. Aerobic adaptations

9. Which of the following is defined as the use of recreating successful athletic events or endeavors within the athlete's mind?
    a. Mental arousal
    b. Mental imagery
    c. Mental stimulation
    d. Mental practice

10. Social acceptance, trophies, awards, and induction into a hall of fame are all examples of which of the following?
    a. Extrinsic motivation
    b. Self-motivation
    c. Intrinsic motivation
    d. Positive self-talk

11. Adaptation that occurs from stress placed on the body is the definition of which of the following?
    a. Specific adaptation syndrome
    b. Acute adaptation syndrome
    c. Exercise resistance syndrome
    d. General adaptation syndrome

12. Which of the following allows relaxation from a muscle contraction?
    a. Sodium is no longer available for contraction
    b. Lack of contractile fibers and relaxation of the neuron
    c. Lack of calcium available and signal cessation from the motor neuron
    d. External resistance overload and Golgi tendon organ activation

13. What is the primary location of hemoglobin?
    a. Lymphocytes
    b. White blood cells
    c. Adrenal glands
    d. Red blood cells

14. Which of the following accurately describes bone periosteum?
    a. Spongy tissue located within the bone matrix
    b. Cells within the bone that bring nutrients to the bone tissue
    c. Specialized bone tissue that connects the bones to tendons
    d. Central location of bone where growth occurs during development

15. Which of the following is NOT considered a form of feedback during instruction?
    a. Augmented feedback
    b. Segmented feedback
    c. Knowledge of results
    d. Knowledge of performance

16. Which of the following accurately describes detraining?
    a. Loss of physical attributes attained from training after a period of inactivity
    b. Performance increases from training at reduced intensities from the initial ones
    c. Adaptation from periods of rest that allow the body to attain performance improvements
    d. Performance increases from normal development rather than from physical training

17. Why will cardiac output increase as the intensity and workload increase within a given submaximal bout of exercise in a trained athlete compared to an untrained athlete?
    a. Heart rate is slower than it would have been previously
    b. The heart is beating faster than it used to at the same workload
    c. Vital organs require more oxygenated blood
    d. Stoke volume increases

18. The joints between the vertebrae of the human body are of which type?
    a. Fibrous Joints
    b. Synovial Joints
    c. Cartilaginous joints
    d. Ball and Socket Joints

19. Which of the following is NOT a recommended guideline when training children and adolescents?
    a. 1RM testing
    b. 1-3 sets of 6-15 repetitions for exercises
    c. Performing an appropriate warm-up
    d. Direct supervision from a qualified strength and conditioning professional

20. Which of the following is defined as administering tasks, objects, or events that would likely decrease the occurrence of a negative operant?
    a. Negative Punishment
    b. Positive Punishment
    c. Negative reinforcement
    d. Positive reinforcement

21. As actin and myosin filaments interact, what occurs to the Z-lines?
    a. Z-lines start to separate
    b. Z-lines begin to move towards each other
    c. Z-lines disappear
    d. Z-lines are unchanged

22. What is the term used for the motor neuron and the muscle fibers it innervates?
    a. Neuromuscular junction
    b. Axon terminal
    c. Motor unit
    d. Myofibril excitation

23. Which of the following is the term used for when the ability of a receptor site to respond to a specific hormone decreases?
    a. Non-responsiveness
    b. Decreased receptor function
    c. Autoregulation
    d. Downregulation

24. Injuries that occur with advanced-aged athletes are due to which of the following?
    a. Loss in neuromotor function
    b. Balance issues
    c. Sarcopenia
    d. Vestibular changes

25. Muscle mass loss that often occurs with older athletes is known as which of the following?
    a. Sarcopenia
    b. Aging muscle loss
    c. Geriatric muscle loss
    d. Atrophy

26. Which of the following is an adaptation of the cardiopulmonary system in response to training?
    a. Decreased oxygen uptake
    b. Vasoconstriction
    c. Decreased maximal heart rate
    d. Increased maximal oxygen uptake

27. Which connective tissue surrounds the individual muscle fibers of the human body?
    a. Epimysium
    b. Fascicles
    c. Endomysium
    d. Perimysium

28. Which of the following is usually best suited for whole practice instruction?
    a. Skills of high complexity but low organization
    b. Skills of low complexity but high organization
    c. Skills of low complexity and organization
    d. Skills of high complexity and organization

29. What muscle fiber type is associated with marathon running?
    a. Type IIx
    b. Type IIa
    c. Type I
    d. Type III

30. What is the term used when a hormone can partially interact with a receptor site?
    a. Hormone partial interaction
    b. Hormone blocking interaction
    c. Partial-reactivity
    d. Cross-reactivity

31. Which of the following accurately describes instructional guided discovery?
    a. Only instructing the athlete on the goal of the task
    b. Giving specific instructions but limiting information to allow athletes to process the movement
    c. Showing an athlete a video of the movement then requiring them to perform the exercise
    d. Instructing the athlete on each specific aspect of the movement and providing feedback along the way

32. Which of the following is a sign of overtraining?
    a. Increases in illness frequency
    b. Increases in muscular flexibility
    c. Decreases in delayed onset muscle soreness
    d. Decreases in resting heart rate

33. During training, removal of an element of the workout that the athlete considers negative represents which of the following reinforcement techniques?
    a. Negative reinforcement
    b. Positive reinforcement
    c. Negative punishment
    d. Positive punishment

34. For exercises that use multiple joints and muscles, such as the Olympic clean and jerk, which of the following instruction modalities have been shown to be the most successful?
    a. Whole practice instruction
    b. Part practice instruction
    c. Sub-part instruction
    d. Comprehensive instruction

35. Which of the following is a disadvantage of using high intensity interval training?
    a. Excessively high heart rates are often experienced
    b. Inappropriate metabolic adaptations can occur
    c. Non-specific movement patterns are reinforced
    d. Stress can rise to counterproductive levels

36. Which of the following is a way that force can be controlled during a muscular contraction?
    a. Activation of actin and myosin
    b. Activation of the motor end plate
    c. Activation of motor units
    d. Activation of an action potential

37. The exchange of inspired air and internal gases is the primary role of which of the following systems?
    a. Lymphatic system
    b. Vascular system
    c. Neuroendocrine system
    d. Respiratory system

38. Which plane is the body moving within during forward lunges?
    a. Transverse plane
    b. Frontal plane
    c. Sagittal Plane
    d. Lateral Plane

39. What is the length that residual effects remain in maximal strength after periods of inactivity?
    a. 5 +/- 5 days
    b. 30 +/- 5 days
    c. 15 +/- 5 days
    d. 18 +/- 4 days

40. Which of the following accurately describes an operant?
    a. A behavior reinforced by a stimulus
    b. The avoidance of a specific behavior
    c. The motivation to avoid a punishment
    d. The motivation to earn a reward

41. During the contraction phase of a dumbbell bent-over row, the latissimus dorsi acts as which of the following?
    a. Synergist
    b. Neutralizer
    c. Agonist
    d. Antagonist

42. Which of the following accurately describes the inverted-U theory?
    a. As the arousal levels rise, performance levels will increase proportionally
    b. Arousal levels increase performance up to an optimal level, but further increases are associated with reduced performance
    c. Arousal levels have no effect on performance and therefore should not be focused on throughout training sessions
    d. As arousal levels decrease, performance increases as the athlete becomes more comfortable and less anxious

43. Where does the electrical impulse for the heart's conduction originate?
    a. AV bundle
    b. Aortic valve
    c. Purkinje fibers
    d. SA node

44. Which of the following relates to the intensity and focus of one's effort?
    a. Motivation
    b. Motive to achieve success
    c. Motive to avoid failure
    d. Reinforcement

45. Which of the following is NOT associated with optimal arousal levels for athletes?
    a. Increased mental activation
    b. Increased performance anxiety
    c. Increased positive thoughts
    d. Increased control in decision-making tasks

46. Which of the following is NOT a strategy used for optimizing hormone levels with training?
    a. Use of multi-joint movements
    b. Use of compound movements
    c. Implementing exercises that use large muscle groups
    d. Focusing on stabilizing muscles

47. Which of the following energy systems is the primary source of ATP generation for the 100-meter dash?
   a. Oxidative
   b. Fast glycolysis
   c. Phosphagen
   d. Slow glycolysis

48. Which of the following is a specific guideline for older adult resistance training?
   a. Static stretching should occur before and after training sessions
   b. Dynamic stretching should occur before and after training sessions
   c. Static stretching should occur before exercise and dynamic stretching should follow after the workout
   d. Dynamic stretching should occur before exercise and static stretching should follow after the workout

49. Which of the following is a common fault when training children and adolescents?
   a. Prescribing individualized programming
   b. Believing the anatomy and physiology are the same as in adults
   c. Prescribing aerobic workloads that are programmed around the specific sport
   d. Spending too much time on instruction and not enough on training

50. A common motive observed in athletes to protect their ego, self-worth, and self-esteem is known as which of the following?
   a. Motive to avoid failure
   b. Motive to achieve success
   c. Motive to protect oneself
   d. Motive to avoid judgement

51. Which of the following is NOT a component of bone?
   a. Calcium carbonate
   b. Calcium phosphate
   c. Sodium bicarbonate
   d. Protein

52. What is the ideal work to rest ratio when trying to train the glycolytic energy system?
   a. 1:12–1:20
   b. 1:15–1:30
   c. 1:1–1:3
   d. 1:3–1:5

53. Which of the following is NOT a primary function of the cardiovascular system?
   a. Exchange of oxygen
   b. Transportation of nutrients
   c. Removal of waste products
   d. Breakdown of nutrients for energy

54. After puberty, which of the following is a common characteristic observed in both males and females?
    a. Equal muscle quality
    b. Equal muscle mass
    c. Equal body fat
    d. Equal flexibility

55. What are the upper limits of "normal" for systolic and diastolic blood pressure?
    a. 120/40 mmHg
    b. 120/80 mmHg
    c. 150/80 mmHg
    d. 150/40 mmHg

56. Which of the following is NOT an adaptation of tendons to exercise training?
    a. Increased fibril diameter
    b. Increased number of cross-links
    c. Increased flexibility
    d. Increased number of connective fibers

57. What is the term used when the body remains in a higher state of oxygen consumption after the cessation of exercise?
    a. Post-exercise oxygen syndrome
    b. Post-exercise increased cardiac output
    c. Excess post-exercise oxygen consumption
    d. Excess post-exercise aerobic capacity

58. Which of the following is NOT considered an anabolic hormone?
    a. Testosterone
    b. Growth hormone
    c. Insulin-like growth factor
    d. Cortisol

59. What is a common hormonal response in males undergoing puberty?
    a. Increase in circulating testosterone
    b. Increase in cortisol at rest
    c. Increase in circulating estrogen
    d. Decrease in growth hormone

Answer Explanations

1. A: When performance begins to decline from stress that is applied to the body throughout training, it is known as function overreaching. Often, functional overreaching is a planned method of increasing stress prior to a period of rest or of reduced intensity. It is important for the strength and conditioning professional to understand a difference between overreaching and overtraining.

2. B: Throughout training, the strength and conditioning professional may instruct the athlete on specific tasks to perform during the movement. This is known as explicit instruction. Explicit instruction can be very beneficial with simple, single-joint, exercises but may be less effective with more advanced, multi-joint, compound movements. Therefore, the strength and conditioning professional should assess the movement category and administer instruction techniques that best suit the exercise, as well as the individual.

3. C: The pectoralis major contracts eccentrically when the barbell is lowered to the chest in a barbell bench press exercise. Almost exclusively, any lowering phase of the external resistance or body will be categorized as an eccentric muscle action of the agonist muscle due to the need to control the downward phase of the movement. Because gravity will cause the load to drop, the muscles must contract eccentrically to control the load. It is important to understand the difference between concentric, eccentric, and isometric muscle actions when designing training protocols for athletes.

4. D: The heart's conduction system can be observed through a graph known as an electrocardiogram. The graph that is displayed during an electrocardiogram is comprised of a P-wave, a QRS complex (Q-wave, R-wave, S-wave), and a T-wave. The P-wave and QRS complex represents the depolarization phase of the atria and ventricles, respectively. The T-wave represents the repolarization phase of contraction.

5. D: During respiration, the lungs expand and retract to control volume of air within the system. The expansion and retraction are controlled by two different mechanisms: the upward and downward movement of the diaphragm and the depression and elevation of the ribs. Although the abdominals can have a role in the expansion and retraction of the lungs, their involvement entails activation and contraction, not active relaxation.

6. B: Attention is the operation of processing environmental, external, and internal cues that enter one's awareness throughout training and competition. It is important for athletes to ensure that their attention and level of focus is based on task-relevant stimuli and keep their attention off of task-irrelevant stimuli.

7. C: For the strength and conditioning professional, it is important to understand the differences between the appendicular and axial skeletons. The axial skeleton consists of the ribs, sternum, vertebral column, and the skull and the appendicular skeleton consists of the bones of the hips, knees, ankles, feet, pelvic girdle, shoulder girdle, arms, wrists, and hands. Acquiring a basic understanding of bone anatomy can be beneficial when speaking with other medical personnel, such as athletic strength and conditioning professionals and team doctors.

8. A: The hormonal response to exercise will not be the same for children and young adolescents as that of the general athletic population. In prepubescent children, circulating hormones such as testosterone, growth hormone, and insulin-like growth factor are limited. Therefore, many of the strength gains afforded from training programs are increased hypertrophy of the musculature and neural adaptations. It is the neural adaptations, including enhanced recruitment of motor units, that primarily drives improvements.

9. B: Mental imagery involves recreating successful athletic events within the mind of the athlete. This recreation can entail every sensory aspect of the event, such as what might be seen, heard, smelled, and felt. By recreating a successful athletic endeavor, the athlete will increase the desire to experience such events within their athletic career again. The mental image does not need to be limited to competition; it may include a successful practice, or rehearsal, in preparation to the event.

10. A: When observing motivation, successful athletes demonstrate both intrinsic and extrinsic motivation. Extrinsic motivation involves the desire for external rewards from successful outcomes of training and competition. Examples include social acceptance, trophies, awards, induction into a hall of fame, and praise. Intrinsic motivation involves the internal desire to be successful, the athlete's love for the sport, and the internal satisfaction gleaned from participation. It is important to note that athletes are usually not solely motivated by extrinsic or intrinsic factors, but from a combination of both.

11. D: Adaptation can occur from any stressor that is placed on the human body, a phenomenon called general adaptation syndrome (GAS). When stress is placed upon the body over time, the body will begin to react accordingly and try to build resistance or tolerance to that stress. In the case of exercise as the stressor, the body adapts by increasing neural recruitment of muscle fibers, increases muscle fiber size and density, increasing mitochondrial density, etc., depending on the specific training program.

12. C: During a muscle contraction, the motor neuron sends an electrical impulse, in the form of an action potential, for the muscle to contract. Furthermore, calcium plays a major role in the interaction. As long as calcium is available, the myosin and actin will continue to interact. When calcium is insufficient or when the action potential ceases, the interaction of the myofibrils will stop and the muscle will relax.

13. D: Hemoglobin is the main vehicle within blood for oxygen transport to the rest of the body. Hemoglobin is located within the red blood cells. As the red blood cells are travel through the bod via the cardiovascular system, the oxygen can reach the cells of the body.

14. C: Almost all bones are surrounded by a specialized tissue called periosteum, which serves as a site for tendon attachment. As muscles contract, tendons, which are connected to bones by the periosteum, pull on the bones, causing movement. Choice *B* is incorrect because although periosteum contains vasculature and nerves, it is not "cells within the bone," but rather an outer coating on the bone made of fibrous tissue.

15. B: Throughout training, especially during learning periods, feedback can have a major impact in eliciting the desired movement patterns. Feedback involves providing the athlete with information about his or her movements patterns or performance of an exercise. This information can then be used to correct any faults in technique or execution. Augmented feedback, knowledge of results, and knowledge of performance are all forms of feedback commonly used in the strength and conditioning profession.

16. A: The decline in fitness gains attained through training after a period of inactivity is called detraining. When the physical stress is removed for an extended period of time, the body responds by regressing back towards an untrained status. The result of this regression is a partial or complete loss of the positive adaptations that resulted in a proper and specific training program.

17. D: Cardiac output is the total volume of blood pumped by the heart. It is a product of the heart rate (how fast the heart is beating) and stroke volume (the volume of blood ejected each beat). Aerobic training can increase both cardiac output and stroke volume. As muscles are performing work, the need for oxygenated blood increases. Therefore, the increase in cardiac output is correlated to the increased intensity and workload of the exercise. Choice *A* is wrong because although a trained athlete should have a slower heart rate for a given submaximal workload, this reduction doesn't explain the reason that cardiac output at that workload is higher in a trained athlete. In fact, since cardiac output is the product of heart rate and stroke volume, a slower heart rate alone would decrease cardiac output. It is because of the much greater stroke volume that cardiac output actually increases despite one factor (heart rate) decreasing. Choice *B* is incorrect because although heart rate increases with higher exercise intensities, a *trained* individual (which was stated in the question) actually experiences a slower heart rate than what would have been experienced in an untrained state due to the improved cardiac efficiency and greater stroke volume.

18. C: The intervertebral disks of the human body are cartilaginous joints that allow limited movement in particular planes.

19. A: When administering training to children and adolescents, guidelines for youth resistance training must be followed. First, the youth athlete must understand the benefits and risks associated with the training program. Throughout training, when performing each exercise, the child should be closely monitored by a strength and conditioning professional at all times and should never be left alone. Prior to training, an appropriate and thorough warm-up should be performed. Children and adolescents do not respond to training as adults do; therefore, the exercise response should be closely monitored. Guidelines for exercise volume is approximately 1-3 sets or 6-15 repetitions at an appropriate weight that can be sustained without compromising form. Although, 1 repetition max testing is often utilized in adult training, children and adolescents need a thorough learning period to learn technique and movement patterns. Therefore, 1 repetition max testing would not be suitable for the youth athlete as it can be highly unsafe.

20. B: Positive punishment and negative punishment are considered reinforcement techniques that are utilized within the strength and conditioning profession. When administering punishment reinforcement techniques, the strength and conditioning professional aims to decrease the occurrence of a given undesirable operant; therefore, decreasing the occurrence of the operant can increase the success of the athlete. Positive punishment relates to administering tasks, objects, or events that would likely decrease the occurrence of the negative operant, such as adding sprints to the end of a practice where athletes were continually goofing around.

21. B: The z-line of a sarcomere is where actin filaments are anchored, and each sarcomere is defined by the bounds of adjacent z-lines. The sliding-filament theory states that as the actin and myosin bind and pull towards one another, the ends z-lines move towards each other as the muscle fiber shortens.

22. C: The motor unit is the term used for the motor neuron and all of the muscle fibers it innervates. When an action potential travels down the motor neuron, as long as it is off sufficient intensity to exceed the minimum threshold, all of the fibers in the motor unit will contract together.

23. D: When a receptor site decreases its ability to respond to a specific hormone or negates the response process altogether, it is known as downregulation of receptor function. Downregulation can greatly alter the sensitivity of the receptor, thereby changing the hormonal response of the human body.

24. A: Neuromotor function begins to decline with age and can be related to many of the injuries sustained in older adults. Injuries such as falls, dislocations, and skeletal fractures become common in the elderly. With these factors in mind, strength and conditioning professionals can safely administer neuromotor facilitating exercises into the training of the aging athlete. Furthermore, the strength and conditioning professional must also follow all guidelines for working with this population.

25. A: The loss in muscle mass that occurs with the aging process is called sarcopenia. While this is a natural process for all aging adults, the process can be slowed in adults who remain active since it is thought to mainly occur because of inactivity. Resistance exercise can help preserve muscle mass and slow the decline in strength. Therefore, it is important for older adults to remain physically active. When muscle mass is lost, muscular strength and power also begins to decline. A muscle's cross-sectional area typically starts reducing after the after the age of 30 and will continue to decline if the athlete does not engage in regular, challenging resistance training.

26. D: The cardiovascular system is afforded many benefits from aerobic training. One of these adaptations is the increase in maximal oxygen uptake to meet the increased demand of the heart and muscles for oxygen. Maximum oxygen uptake is a product of cardiac output and the arteriovenous difference, which is a measure of how well the tissues extract oxygen from the circulating blood.

27. C: The endomysium surrounds each individual muscle fiber. Fibers are bundled into fascicles, which have a connective tissue covering called the perimysium. Multiple fascicles are grouped together to form the entire muscle, which is covered in the epimysium.

28. B: Whole practice instruction teaches movements in their entirety. When whole practice teaching occurs, the movements are taught in one fluid movement. Whole practice instruction is best suited for skills that are of low complexity but high organization. Skill complexity relates to the number of components or parts of the task, such that a task of low complexity has just a couple parts whereas one of high complexity has many. A skill that has a higher degree of complexity requires more mental processing to execute, and thus carries a greater cognitive demand. Skill organization the degree to which the components of the skill are spatially and temporally interrelated. Those that are highly interdependent have high levels organization. A cartwheel is an example of a skill best taught using whole practice. Choice *A*, skills of high complexity but low organization, are served well by part practice.

29. C: Type I fibers are classified as slow-twitch muscle fibers and are most suitable for a marathon runner. Type II and Type IIx are both fast-twitch muscle fibers and are more conducive to explosive sporting activities. Type I fibers are efficient muscle fibers that are relatively fatigue-resistant and primarily rely on oxidative pathways for energy production, making them the ideal muscle fiber for a marathon runner.

30. D: When a hormone has the ability to partially interact with a receptor site, it blocks any other interaction from occurring at that site in a process termed cross-reactivity.

31. B: Guided discovery is the term used when specific instructions are given during the learning process but information is limited to allow the athlete to process the movement. Since one of the main drawbacks of explicit instruction is "information overload," guided discovery gives the athlete the main information of the movement, but allows him or her to learn certain aspects independently as the movement is performed. The information given during guided discovery often relates to preventing injury during the movement, but the remaining information is left for the athlete to discover. This technique also allows the athlete to process new material at his or her own pace and connect more strongly with internal cues.

32. A: There are a variety of signs of overtraining. One of the main signs is poorer immunity, which manifests as more frequent sickness or illness. When the stress of training is too significant or constant without ample recovery, the immune system becomes depressed and less able to fend off illnesses. Other symptoms of overtraining can include muscle stiffness and soreness, difficulty sleeping, mood and appetite changes, and an increase in resting heart rate.

33. A: Negative reinforcement involves the removal of a certain element that the athlete views negatively. An example of using this technique is if an athlete completes the workout with a great attitude and demonstrates leadership, then he or she wouldn't have to perform the resisted runs at the end. By removing the negative element (difficult resisted runs), the probability of the operant occurring again might increase.

34. B: For complex movements that require use of multiple muscle groups and joints, part practice instruction may be more conducive to skill acquisition. In part practice instruction, each segment of the movement can be broken down in subcomponents to ensure each segment is taught prior to performing the movement as a whole. Skills of high complexity but low organization are served well by part practice. Skill complexity relates to the number of components or parts of the task, such that a task of low complexity has just a couple parts whereas one of high complexity has many. A skill that has a higher degree of complexity requires more mental processing to execute, and thus carries a greater cognitive demand. Skill organization the degree to which the components of the skill are spatially and temporally interrelated. Those that are highly interdependent have high levels organization. A backflip is an example of a skill for which part practice might be beneficial. The coach could first teach a handstand, then bending into a bridge, then kicking up back out of the bridge.

35. D: High Intensity Interval Training (HIIT) is a variation of interval training that incorporates intermittent rest periods and repeated bouts of intense work. This can be very useful workout when time is limited in a session but a strong metabolic conditioning stimulus is desired. Running, cycling, and jump roping are often modes of exercises used in HIIT training. When used properly, HIIT has the ability to produce advantageous adaptations to metabolic, neuromuscular, and cardiopulmonary systems simultaneously. Although there are many advantages to HIIT, one must be cautious when using HIIT concurrently with other means of athletic development. HIIT can be very stressful on the body and can result in a higher incidence of injury or overtraining. Therefore, one of the major drawbacks of high intensity interval training is that stress can rise to counterproductive levels.

36. C: During training and daily life, the body can moderate the force of muscular contractions in two primary ways. The first is through the frequency of activation of the motor units. If a motor unit is only activated once, then a twitch will result and the force will be low. As more action potentials are fired, twitches begin to overlap and summate, and the force of the contraction will increase. The second way the body can control the force of a contraction is through recruitment, which involves altering the number of motor units stimulated. Through the recruitment strategy, the body and brain can detect how many motor units are required for a given activity, as well as what type of fibers are needed for the activity and then send action potentials to those motor neurons accordingly.

37. D: The respiratory system allows for the cells and tissues of the body to receive oxygen and remove carbon dioxide through the process of breathing.

38. C: Understanding the planes in which the body moves can be very beneficial when communicating with other medical personnel such as athletic strength and conditioning professionals and team doctors. Therefore, the strength and conditioning professional must acquire knowledge of the movement planes of the human body. When performing a forward lunge, the movement is occurring within the sagittal plane because there is forward flexion and extension of the hips, knees, and ankles and the body is moving forward when visualized from the side.

39. B: When considering detraining effects, it is important to understand the length of time that residual effect gained during programming will last for each athletic attribute. For maximal strength, residual effects tend to remain 30 days, plus or minus 5 days, until regression occurs.

40. A: An *operant* is a specific outcome that is targeted through stimulus conditioning, though it is not initially the result of a specific stimulus; instead, at first, it is a behavior that occurs spontaneously. It is through the different reinforcing or deterring techniques (or consequences from the operant) that the operant becomes the targeted outcome of a stimulus. Four different reinforcement techniques can be used to reinforce the operant and increase the probability of its occurrence. These techniques are positive reinforcement, negative reinforcement, positive punishment, and negative punishment.

41. C: The prime mover in any exercise is known as the agonist. Therefore, the agonist during the dumbbell bent-over row, is the latissimus dorsi, since it is one of the prime movers for the exercise.

42. B: Although higher arousal levels are associated with higher performance outcomes, heightened arousal states are finite and can become detrimental if the arousal level becomes too high. The inverted-U theory describes this phenomenon. It states that arousal levels up to a certain level increase performance, but further increases in arousal are associated with reduced performance.

43. D: The heart's electrical impulse originates in the SA node, which is considered the intrinsic pacemaker of the heart. It then travels to the AV node and then onward. This conduction system is what stimulates the heart to contract and maintain its rhythm.

44. A: The intensity and focus of one's effort is a product of motivation. Motivation for competition and training, as well as a desire to be successful, can have major implications to the outcome of one's athletic career. Successful athletes usually possess a combination of both intrinsic and extrinsic motivation.

45. B: Optimal arousal levels are very important in attaining success in athletics. Being able to achieve optimal arousal levels can have a major impact on the outcome and performance of an athletic event. When optimal arousal levels are achieved, increases can be seen in mental activation, positive self-thoughts, and decision-making tasks. Although performance anxiety can be associated with arousal levels, this problem is often observed when the arousal levels rise too high, so they are no longer "optimal."

46. D: When trying to achieve the optimal hormonal response to training, the strength and conditioning professional should be knowledgeable about the exercises that elicit such responses. Using ground-based, multi-joint movements, as well as those that use large muscle groups, can increase blood concentrations of the anabolic hormones such as testosterone and growth hormone. Therefore, the strength and conditioning professional should incorporate exercises such as deadlifts, squats, power cleans, front squats, and Romanian deadlifts into all training programs that are geared toward increasing muscle strength and size.

47. C: The phosphagen system is the primary energy system used in the beginning of movement and when ATP must be generated extremely quickly during short-duration exercise of a very high intensity. This system has a small amount of ATP readily available, which is why it is exhausted first during exercise. It also can generate a small amount of ATP very quickly since the energy-generation pathway is so short, so it is the system of choice for high-intensity activities lasting about 10-seconds or less.

48. D: There are many guidelines to follow when administering resistance training to older adults. One of these guidelines involves stretching to increase flexibility. It is always advisable to do a thorough warm-up with dynamic stretching prior to a workout and follow the session with static stretching for all of the major muscle groups.

49. B: A lack of understanding of safe youth resistance training is unfortunately common in the strength and conditioning profession. Too often, children and adolescents are treated as adults in terms of programming and exercise selection. Responses to resistance training are different between adults and children because of the differences in anatomy and physiology, particularly the immature skeleton and prepubescent hormonal profile of the child. These differences need to be considered when designing programs for youth athletes.

50. A: Motive to avoid failure is a motive for the athlete to protect their ego, self-worth, and self-esteem. It is important to note that a motive to avoid failure is not to avoid failure per se, but to avoid the perception of shame from one's team, coaches, fans, and family. Athletes with a high motive to avoid failure tend to seek out competitions that are easy and unchallenging to them personally.

51. C: Basic bone anatomy consists of non-living minerals as well as living bone cells. Bone is primarily made of calcium carbonate, calcium phosphate, and the protein called collagen. Sodium bicarbonate is not a foundational element of bone.

52. D: When designing activities specific to the energy system of the sporting activity, work-to-rest ratios become vitally important. The work-to-rest ratio is the amount of predetermined time for the exercise to occur (work period) to the length of time exercise should cease (rest). Work-to-rest ratios for the glycolytic energy system are approximately 1:3–1:5.

53. D: The strength and conditioning professional must understand the structure and function of the cardiovascular system and how it responds to the training process. Primarily, the cardiovascular system is responsible for the transporting oxygen and nutrients throughout the body and delivering it to the cells and tissues for use and removing waste from the cells, such as carbon dioxide. The breakdown of nutrients for energy is a function of the digestive system, not the cardiovascular system.

54. A: Although after puberty males generally have more muscle mass than females, the quality of muscle tissue itself tends to be the same in both sexes. The greater strength and power typically seen in males is due to the increased muscle mass itself and not from a higher quality tissue.

55. B: Understanding normal blood pressure is beneficial to the strength and conditioning professional because it can help the strength and conditioning professional spot dangerous, hypertensive levels and refer the patient to an appropriate medical provider. The upper limits of normal blood pressure as of November 2017 are 120/80. Although hypertension used to be considered defined as a blood pressure of greater than or equal to 140/90 mmHg, it is now defined as ≥130/80 mm Hg.

56. C: Since muscles and bones both adapt to external resistance, the tendons and ligaments of the body must do the same to withstand the loads that the muscle and bone can now produce and accommodate. Adaptations of the tendons to through the training process to withstand greater loads include increasing fibril diameter, forming more cross-linkages, and the developing new collagen fibers. They do not usually become more flexible; in fact, the adaptations tend to make them stiffer, which is also advantageous for a higher rate of energy return.

57. C: During exercise, especially at higher intensities, the body uses an excessive amount of oxygen to fuel the working muscles and heart. Once the bout of exercise stops, oxygen uptake remains elevated over baseline levels, which is termed excess post-exercise oxygen consumption (EPOC). The function of EPOC is to help restore homeostasis in the different systems of the body that were active during the workload period. exercise.

58. D: During the training process, adaptations can occur from the release and storage of certain hormones that promote tissue building. Hormones that promote the tissue building process, especially during protein synthesis, are termed anabolic hormones. Anabolic hormones include testosterone, insulin, and insulin-like growth factor. Cortisol is a catabolic hormone because it signals the body to break down tissues.

59. A: As males undergo puberty, an increase in testosterone can be observed. This increase in testosterone is responsible for increases in muscle mass and bone formation observed during and after puberty.

Nutrition

Nutrition can have a major impact on an athlete's training, performance, physiology, injury risk, hormonal balance, mood, and body composition. Therefore, strength and conditioning professionals need to have a thorough understanding of at least the foundations of nutrition for health and performance to help provide information and guidance to athletes and identify issues that necessitate a referral to an appropriate professional such as a registered dietician or team doctor. The following sections provide basic nutrition information and ways to appropriately apply this information within the strength and conditioning profession.

Nutritional Factors Affecting Health and Performance

Athletes and physically active individuals require extra calories and certain nutrients to fuel their energy expenditure and prepare and replenish the bod for training and competitions. Therefore, the strength and conditioning professional must understand many nutritional factors that affect the general health and physical performance of the athlete. These factors include nutrition science, nutritional needs of different athletes based on individuality and sport, health risks associated with certain nutrient deficits or excesses, proper hydration requirements, and ideal dietary intake in terms of foods and timing.

Health-Related and Performance-Related Application of Nutritional Concepts

On many occasions, athletes may ask their strength and conditioning coach for nutritional advice for both health and performance. Educating athletes in proper health and performance nutrition is important but can be enhanced if the athlete has a basic understanding of nutrition parameters. MyPlate can be a valuable tool to help athletes learn about their fundamental nutritional needs. MyPlate is a dietary intake guidance tool issued by the United States Department of Agriculture and can help individuals understand their basic nutritional needs based on their age, sex, and physical activity. It is important to note that many of the recommendations are based on the needs of the general population and may need adjustment to accommodate the increased nutritional needs that athletes often require for optimal performance and health.

That said, MyPlate is a good starting point for relatively healthy athletes to evaluate their current diet and identify areas of their diet that are inadequate or not ideal. Therefore, the strength and conditioning professional should have a good understanding of MyPlate and how to modify the recommendations to accommodate the nutritional needs associated with optimal performance and health. MyPlate categorizes food groups into five main groups: fruits, vegetables, grains, protein, and dairy. Although the recommended serving for each group is given for general population and not competitive athletes, the actual food groups do coincide with a diet conducive to good health and even performance. Therefore, the same food groups should be incorporated into the diet of all athletes, although the serving sizes may need to be adjusted.

When evaluating an athlete's diet, it is important to ensure that a variety of macronutrients (carbohydrates, fats, and protein) and micronutrients (vitamins and minerals) are consumed. Athletes a generalization, many athletes tend to avoid change and have certain routines set that they believe enhance their performance. Therefore, it can be challenging to modify an athlete's dietary consumption unless he or she is eager and open to change. It is important to encourage athletes to change their consumption of each food group, where appropriate, to better align with their needs and the recommendations set forth by respected nutrition resources such as the United States Department of

Agriculture. Explaining the benefits of the suggested modifications can help facilitate the adjustment. Athletes, in particular, should strive to have diets with a lot of variety of foods within each category to provide a wide array of micronutrients. For example, using the fruit category as an example, an athlete that eats an apple a day, every day, will be consuming fewer micronutrients than an athlete that eats an apple on Monday, a banana on Tuesday, a pear on Wednesday, grapes on Thursday, and an orange on Friday. By consuming different fruits, the athlete can better ensure that most micronutrients, found in fruit, will be consumed throughout the week. Often, a dislike of the taste or texture is the reason for not eating a certain food. Therefore, the strength and conditioning professional should understand the macronutrient and micronutrient breakdown of many foods to offer alternative suggestions of foods with similar nutrients but different flavors. The interchanging of foods with similar nutrient profiles is referred to as a *food exchange* and can greatly enhance the compliance of athletes when giving nutritional advice.

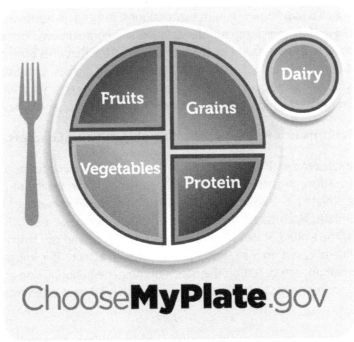

Grains	Vegetables	Fruit
Whole-grain bread	Broccoli	Berries
Cereal	Mushrooms	Melon
Oats	Asparagus	Oranges
Corn Tortillas	Spinach	Apples
	Pumpkin	Pears
	Squash	Kiwi

Dairy	Protein	
Milk	Chicken	Tofu
Cheese	Turkey	Legumes
Yogurt,	Fish	Egg
Cottage Cheese	Lean Beef	Seeds

Once an athlete has an established diet based on optimal performance and health, the glycemic index and load should be evaluated. *Glycemic index* refers to a ranking system based on how quickly carbohydrates are digested, absorbed, and used as fuel. By tracking the glycemic index, the athlete can monitor the rate of increase on blood glucose levels within a two-hour time frame after consumption. Food groups with lower glycemic indexes are digested and absorbed slower than those with a higher glycemic index.

Nutritional Needs for Various Athletes for Carbohydrates, Protein, Fat, Vitamins, and Minerals

Nutritional needs will vary widely depending on the sport and performance goals of the athlete. Too often, strength and conditioning professionals assume that a certain diet will work for many different athletes. Athletes, and their bodies, need individualized nutritional protocols that are based around the sporting activity, training intensity, personal preferences, body composition, and health status of the athlete. The following provides generalized guidelines to use as a starting point when developing individualized nutrition programs for athletes:

Aerobic Endurance Nutrition
- Consume 8 to 10 grams of carbohydrates per kilogram of body weight
- Consume 1 to 1.6 grams of protein per kilogram of body weight
- Increase of sodium and potassium for prolonged activity
- Consume a low to moderate intake of healthy fats

Strength Sport Nutrition
- Consume 5 to 6 grams of carbohydrates per kilogram of body weight to minimize muscular breakdown

- Consume 1.4 to 1.7 grams of protein per kilogram of body weight

- Consume a moderate amount of fat from healthy sources to support hormonal balance

- Consume 30 to 100 grams of higher-glycemic carbohydrates post-exercise, especially exercise that causes muscle damage

- Increase of leucine-containing protein

Caloric Needs for Athletes Based on Activity Levels
Males:
- Light activity: 17 kilocalories per pound of body weight or 38 kilocalories per kilogram of body weight

- Moderate activity: 19 kilocalories per pound of body weight or 41 kilocalories per kilogram of body weight

- Heavy activity: 23 kilocalories per pound of body weight or 50 kilocalories per kilogram of body weight

Females:

- Light activity: 16 kilocalories per pound of body weight or 35 kilocalories per kilogram of body weight

- Moderate activity: 17 kilocalories per pound of body weight or 37 kilocalories per kilogram of body weight

- Heavy activity: 20 kilocalories per pound of body weight or 44 kilocalories per kilogram of body weight

Taking these guidelines into account, as well as the components from MyPlate, can ensure athletes are well nourished for competition and training. It is important to note that although the strength and conditioning professional should be knowledgeable about the nutritional needs of athletes, he or she should refer the athlete to a professional for more in-depth nutritional advice.

Health Risk Factors Associated With Dietary Choices

Nutrition can play a major role in development of health risks within every population. Since athletes usually have higher caloric needs, these health risks can increase if regular monitoring is not performed. Therefore, the strength and conditioning professional must take proper steps to ensure that caloric and nutritional requirements are met but not exceeded. Again, it is important to refer the athlete to a dedicated nutrition professional when his or her nutritional needs or concerns are more in depth or if the strength and conditioning professional feels the needed advice exceeds his or her scope of practice.

In terms of macronutrients, fat is the most concerning when evaluating the health risks associated with higher caloric needs. Higher fat intake can increase circulating cholesterol levels. Cholesterol is a viscous, fatty substance that has many functions, such as serving a critical role in plasma membrane formation and building sex hormones. Although these functions are necessary for optimal performance and health, hypercholesteremia (both in terms of total cholesterol and especially high levels of low-density lipoproteins) and high triglycerides are associated with a heightened risk of heart disease and stroke. Normal ranges for total cholesterol are those less than 200 milligrams per deciliter, and for low-density lipoprotein, normal ranges are those below 100 milligrams per deciliter. One of the main nutritional interventions that can be used by the strength and conditioning professional is to monitor the saturated fat intake of the athlete. Saturated fat can increase low-density lipoprotein, thus increasing the risk for heart disease and stroke. In reality, the body can make saturated fat on its own, and no dietary consumption of saturated fat is needed.

The other major concern in terms of macronutrients is the type and quality of carbohydrate intake. Excessive refined, simple sugars, like those found in sodas, cookies, candies, and many processed foods, have been shown to contribute to the risk for heart disease, stroke, metabolic syndrome, and type 2 diabetes. While carbohydrate consumption is important for active individuals, the sources should center around whole, unprocessed foods with fiber like whole grains and vegetables.

For micronutrients, low levels of iron and calcium can cause health risks within the athletic population. Iron is required for hemoglobin synthesis and oxygen transport within the blood since hemoglobin brings oxygen to the cells of the body via the circulatory system. More specifically, iron is a main component of myoglobin, which brings oxygen to muscles. With this information, it is easy to see the need for iron in the nutritional program of an athlete. Low iron levels occur in three different stages: depletion, marginal deficiency, and anemia. When anemia occurs for a prolonged period, red blood cells stop being produced, which limits the amount of oxygen that is transported around the body. Low iron levels can cause fatigue, poor concentration, weakness, decreased exercise and work capacity, and a dry mouth. Each of these symptoms can greatly decrease the performance of an athlete. Therefore, the strength and conditioning professional should ensure enough iron-rich food groups are being consumed each day. Iron within food is divided into two categories: heme and nonheme iron sources. Heme iron sources are those found in animal-derived sources such as red meat, fish, and poultry. Nonheme iron sources are those found in fruits, vegetables, grains, and iron-fortified breakfast cereals. Heme iron sources are more beneficial than nonheme iron sources, since nonheme iron sources are less absorbable in the body. When nonheme iron sources are consumed, only 2 to 20 percent of the iron is bioavailable; therefore, the strength and conditioning professional should ensure that animal-based protein sources rich in iron are consumed unless the vegetarian athlete is very cognizant of his or her need for extra iron. Lastly, if the nutritional needs cannot be met through whole foods, the athlete may need to look into an iron supplement.

For optimal performance and health, adequate calcium intake is also crucial. Calcium helps maintain bone density, which is imperative for preventing stress-related injuries in high-impact sports. When dietary calcium in inadequate, calcium is pulled from bones and to supply the immediate needs to the muscles, blood, and intracellular fluids. When this occurs, bone density decreases and the risk of fractures increases, especially later in life since bone mineral depletion can be difficult to reverse and naturally occurs after the age of 25 or 30 anyway. Therefore, the strength and conditioning professional should ensure that calcium levels are met through a balanced diet. Food sources such as cheese, sardines, cottage cheese, milk, kale, and calcium-fortified orange juice are all sources that can be suggested, among many others.

Effects of Hydration Status and Electrolyte Balance/Imbalance on Health and Performance

Between 45 and 75 percent of the human body is water. With at least half the body consisting of water, proper hydration status is imperative to optimal performance. Therefore, the strength and conditioning professional must understand proper hydration techniques as well as electrolyte balance.

Hydration
For athletes, proper hydration is critical to optimal performance and recovery. With the amount of sweat lost in training and competition, hydration status can quickly become compromised. This compromised state, known as a *hypohydrated state,* causes an increase in core body temperature, a decrease in blood plasma levels, an increase in perceived exertion, and an increase in heart rate. Each of these can become detrimental to athletic performance and daily function. When the hypohydrated state is not rectified, the athlete can become dehydrated. Dehydration can further increase the risks of hypohydration, and lengthen the time needed to regain the proper hydration status. Mild dehydration, even at 2 percent of total body weight, has been shown to have negative effects on athletic performance, including increased fatigue, little-to-no motivation for training and competition, a decrease in power and strength, and a decrease in neuromuscular control, which can increase injury risk.

To prevent or combat hypohydration or dehydration, the strength and conditioning professional must require athletes to adhere to an individualized hydration plan. To begin the development of this plan, the urine specific gravity (USG) test can be used to initially assess the current hydration status of the athlete. The USG will give the strength and conditioning professional a chronic hydration profile that is resistant to acute changes. Therefore, this test is a great tool when assessing the hydration status of any athlete. Once the current hydration status is identified, daily weigh-ins can be conducted. By weighing the athlete pre- and post-training, the strength and conditioning professional can determine hydration needs based on the amount of fluid lost (as detected by weight changes) after workouts.

Electrolytes

Electrolyte imbalances can have negative implications on health and performance. Therefore, the electrolytes lost in sweat need to be considered when devising individualized hydration plans for athletes. The primary electrolytes to consider replacing are sodium, chloride, potassium, magnesium, and calcium. It is important to note that sodium plays a major role in fluid regulation by helping retain fluids when consumed. Therefore, the strength and conditioning professional should ensure enough sodium is consumed through food or drink both during activity and daily life. Different strategies can be used to ensure proper electrolyte balance is met. Increasing dietary sodium intake, consuming electrolyte-containing sports drinks, and the adding electrolyte supplements to drinking water can help an athlete maintain an adequate electrolyte balance.

Caloric- Versus Nutrient-Dense Foods

When designing individual nutrition and hydration plans for athletes, it is important to explain the difference between calorically-dense and nutrient-dense foods. Calorically-dense foods are foods that do not have much nutritional value but contain a lot of calories. Examples are desserts, cookies, potato chips, candy, and soda. Nutrient-dense foods are foods that have many micronutrients and macronutrients. Examples of nutrient-dense foods are fruits, vegetables, eggs, legumes, fish, and lean meats.

When athletes are encouraged to increase their caloric intake, it is important to ensure that quality calories are added. Nutrient-dense foods should be chosen over calorically-dense foods to ensure the quality of the diet does not suffer and that nutritional needs are met.

Manipulating Food Choices and Training Methods to Maximize Performance

Training and Nutritional Programs That Produce Specific Changes in Body Composition

Being equipped with the proper knowledge in fat loss and lean mass increase is very important for the strength and conditioning professional. Many occasions arise when athletes are not feeling they are performing at optimal levels, and the decrease in performance is due to issues with body size and composition. Although the effects of a proper nutrition program will greatly affect one's body size and composition, principles within the training program can also enhance the body adaptations. To modify the calorie consumption of an athlete, the strength and conditioning professional should first calculate the athlete's basal metabolic rate (BMR). BMR calculates the number of calories needed for the body to function at rest. After the BMR is determined, calorie needs are increased to accommodate the energy needed for activities such as training and ADLs (activities of daily living). Once the BMR and activity energy expenditure are calculated, the strength and conditioning professional can start determining nutritional suggestions in accordance with the specific goals of the athlete.

Fat Loss

Fat loss is often a goal for athletes because it can often improve athletic ability, as long as the athlete indeed has excessive body fat and goes about losing it in a healthy way. Generally, for fat loss to occur, energy expenditure needs to exceed energy consumption. Two main factors that dictate the success of nutrition programs aimed at fat loss are total caloric intake and adherence to the prescribed diet.

For calorie restriction, athletes should strive for a maximum of an intake deficit of around 500 calories per day. By just moderately reducing calories, the athlete will be in a slight energy deficit but not be too depleted as to experience adverse effects especially in terms of performance declines. Maintaining a deficit of roughly 500 calories per day will equate to a weight loss of around one pound of body fat per week. To maintain muscle during the fat loss period, protein intake should be increased to encourage muscle repair and synthesis. Protein should be increased to 1.8 to 2.7 grams of protein per kilogram of body weight. Adherence to the diet is also very important. A diet that is not consistently followed will not be as successful as a one that is followed precisely. When creating a nutrition program for fat loss, the strength and conditioning professional should meet with the athlete to ensure nutrient needs are attained in the diet, especially when the total number of calories are lowered. Adherence in the initial implementation phase of the program can greatly improve the success of the program.

When designing training programs to encourage a reduction in body fat, aerobic activities should be included to increase the daily energy expenditure. Although other training means should still be incorporated, aerobic activities and metabolic conditioning exercises like interval training have been shown to result in the greatest energy expenditures. When designing these fat loss training programs, it is important to monitor the central nervous system, as well as the athlete as a whole, to prevent overtraining. The energy demands of the exercise, coupled with the caloric restriction from the diet, can have detrimental effects on the athlete if he or she is not carefully monitored.

Increase in Lean Body Mass

Athletes are ever-increasing in size and strength. Therefore, many athletes strive to increase their lean body mass to further improve their athletic performance. Through proper nutritional strategies, increases in lean body mass can give the athletes the ability to move more efficiently and with more power. Although daily caloric intake must increase to increase lean body mass, weight gain and body composition should be monitored to ensure the athlete is primarily gaining lean muscle mass. The quality of mass increase, be it adipose or muscle tissue, will greatly affect athletic performance.

When attempting to increase lean body mass, an athlete should consume around 500 additional calories per day than his or her needs. Bumping up intake more drastically can result in fat gain. When designing an individualized nutrition program that increases daily caloric intake, the strength and conditioning professional should incorporate three different strategies that have proven successful in attaining this goal: require the athlete to eat larger portion sizes, increase the athlete's meal frequency, and focus on foods that are more calorie dense. Also, when attempting to increase lean body mass, athletes should increase their consumption of protein. This protein consumption be between 1.5 and 2 grams per kilogram of body weight. Lastly, athletes could consider supplementation of creatine monohydrate. Creatine monohydrate supplementation in a dose of 5 grams has been shown effective in safely and efficiently increasing an athlete's lean body mass.

Composition and Timing of Nutrient and Fluid Intake Before, During, and After an Exercise Session or Sport Event

Nutrient and fluid timing can have a major impact on the outcome of the exercise training session or sporting activity. Therefore, the strength and conditioning professional should acquire a thorough understanding of what food choices are conducive to optimal performance. Since different training activities and sports use different energy systems for the demands placed on the body, nutritional strategies should be programmed around the energy demands of the activity. Also, the nutritional needs vary between pre-competition, during competition, and post-competition time periods. The following provides information for the composition and timing of nutrient and fluid intake during each phase.

Pre-Competition Nutrition

The goals of pre-competition nutrition are to maintain and increase the hydration status of the individual and increase carbohydrate intake to maximize blood glucose and stored glycogen levels. Since dehydration has many ill effects on performance, athletes should maintain hydration status leading up to a sporting event or training activity. Hydration needs may rise when many of the body functions increase in activity prior to competition due to pre-competition nerves or excitement. Furthermore, carbohydrate consumption is very important in pre-competition nutrition, since glycogen is the primary fuel source for most training and sporting activities.

For nutrition consumption occurring four or more hours prior to the training activity or sporting event, athletes should consume specific amounts of carbohydrates and fluids in a balanced meal containing protein and healthy fats. Carbohydrate consumption, during this period, should consist of 1 to 4 grams of carbohydrates per kilogram of body weight. Protein consumption is less important at this time but should still be included. The protein consumption range is between 0.15 and 0.25 grams of protein per kilogram of body weight. Lastly, fats should be included but limited to healthy and natural sources, which may or may not be included within the carbohydrate and protein sources of the meal. For fluid intake, the athlete should consume 5 to 7 milliliters of water per kilogram of body weight. Sports drinks that consist of electrolytes, sodium, and potassium could also be substituted for water at this time.

As the start time for the exercise approaches, the athlete's nutritional needs will vary slightly. For nutritional consumption occurring two hours prior to competition, athletes should consume 1 gram of carbohydrates per kilogram of body weight. Other macronutrient consumption of protein and fats will become less important and should be in trace forms of the carbohydrate-driven meal. During this time, the athlete should continually sip on water or a sports drink to prevent excessive urination while still consuming fluids. The athlete should consume 3 to 5 milliliters, or 10 to 17 ounces, of fluids during this time.

Lastly, within the hour leading up to the training activity or sporting event, the athlete should consume 0.5 grams of carbohydrates per kilogram of body weight, and fluids should be sipped continually, as needed, but not excessively. By incorporating the previous nutritional strategies, the strength and conditioning professional can help ensure that the athlete's blood glucose, glycogen stores, and hydration status are adequate for optimal performance.

During-Event Nutrition
Athletes are often not afforded the opportunity to properly replenish lost energy during a sporting competition. Although this is not optimal, the strength and conditioning professional must take advantage of any opportunities that arise during the course of a competition to rehydrate and refuel. Many of the nutrients lost during competition are in the form of stored muscle and liver glycogen, water, and micronutrients, specifically sodium and potassium. It should also be noted that weather and relative humidity will also play a major role in the nutrients lost during competition. Hotter climates will require more deliberate intervention to maintain adequate nutrient stores throughout exercise. During times of nutrient loss, sodium should be consumed in the range of 460 to 690 milligrams per liter, and potassium should be within the range of 80 to 195 milligrams per liter. To increase blood glucose and glycogen stores, athletes should consume multiple types of carbohydrates such as maltodextrin, glucose, fructose, and sucrose.

Post-competition Nutrition
Post-competition nutrition will be focused on three main primary goals: repairing muscle tissue, rehydration, and replenishing glycogen stores. When developing a post-competition dietary protocol, the strength and conditioning professional must consider the sporting activity, and the athlete's amount of playing time, weight, age, and sex.

For micronutrients, loss of fluids and electrolytes is usually observed after competition. Therefore, athletes should start drinking fluids immediately after competition to replenish the fluid lost. Sports drinks and water should be encouraged. Furthermore, sodium and potassium should be consumed. Lightly salted post-competition foods and natural forms of potassium, such as bananas, should be encouraged.

For macronutrients, natural forms of protein and carbohydrates should be encouraged. If needed, a post-competition protein supplement can be consumed. The following provides information on the protein needs of athletes in the post-competition state:

- Low- to moderate-intensity sporting activity: 0.2 to 0.5 grams per kilogram of body weight
- Elite endurance or high-intensity sporting activity: 0.2 to 0.5 grams per kilogram of body weight
- American football: 20 to 25 grams of high-quality protein
- Olympic weight lifting: 20 to 25 grams of egg/whey protein blend

Carbohydrates should also be consumed after muscle-damaging training and post competition. The amount of carbohydrates will depend on the activity and the intensity at which the activity took place. For example, for aerobic endurance sporting activities, 1.5 grams of carbohydrates per kilogram of body weight are recommended while for strength and power sporting activities, 30 to 100 grams total of high-glycemic carbohydrates are recommended.

Nutritional Factors That Affect Muscular Endurance, Hypertrophy, Strength, and Aerobic Endurance

As previously stated, many nutritional factors will influence the training adaptations that occur throughout the training cycle. Incorporating the proper nutritional strategies based on sport and activity will greatly affect the outcomes of the adaptations. Therefore, the strength and conditioning professional should have a basic understanding of the nutritional components that should be incorporated to positively affect the various performance goals of the athlete. The following provides further information on the specific components in nutritional strategies based around the performance goals of the athlete.

Aerobic Endurance Nutrition
- Consume 8 to 10 grams of carbohydrates per kilogram of body weight daily.

- Consume 1 to 1.6 grams of protein per kilogram of body weight daily.

- Pre-competition meals should consist of 1 to 4 grams of carbohydrates per kilogram of body weight as long as the activity is at least four hours away. Pre-competition meals that are consumed within two hours should include 1 gram of carbohydrates per kilogram of body weight.

- Increase sodium and potassium for prolonged activities.

- Consume 28 to 144 grams of carbohydrates (in the form of sucrose, glucose, maltodextrin, and fructose) per hour during prolonged activities to combat exhaustion.

- Consume a low to moderate intake of healthy fats.

- Consume 1.5 grams of carbohydrates per kilogram of body weight and at least 10 grams of protein post-exercise.

- Focus on replenishing glycogen stores throughout the day to prepare for the next training bout or competition.

Strength Sport Nutrition
- Consume 5 to 6 grams of carbohydrates per kilogram of body weight to minimize muscular breakdown.

- Supplement with carbohydrates before and during training and competition to minimize muscle breakdown.

- Consume 30 to 100 grams of higher-glycemic carbohydrates post-exercise, especially with exercises that cause muscle damage.

- Consume 1.4 to 1.7 grams of protein per kilogram of body weight.

- Younger athletes (up to age 16 or so) should consume 20 to 25 grams of protein post workout, whereas older athletes should consume 40 grams or more to maximize protein synthesis.

- Consume a moderate amount of fat from healthy sources to encourage hormonal balance throughout competition and training.

- Increase of leucine-containing protein.

Nutrition for Hypertrophy
- Consume 30 to 100 grams of higher-glycemic carbohydrates after muscle-damaging activities to reduce the amount of muscle protein breakdown.

- Younger athletes (under age 16 or so) should consume 20 to 25 grams of protein post-workout, whereas older athletes should consume 40 grams or more to maximize protein synthesis.

- Consume meals that contain at least 20 to 30 grams of high-leucine protein every three to four hours throughout the day.

Nutrition for Muscular Endurance
- Focus on adequate hydration to prevent water weight loss that exceeds 2 percent of body weight.

- Consume a carbohydrate-electrolyte beverage during competition and prolonged exercise to delay fatigue and increase performance.

- Fully replenish glycogen stores prior to next competition or training activity

- Consume protein after training and competitions to minimize soreness and muscular damage.

Signs, Symptoms, and Behaviors Associated with Eating Disorders and Altered Eating Habits

Signs and Symptoms Associated with Disordered Eating, Anorexia, and Bulimia

Strength and conditioning professionals must be aware of the signs, symptoms, and behaviors associated with eating disorders. Eating disorders such as anorexia nervosa and bulimia nervosa are serious mental health disorders that can have dangerous side effects and, in serious cases, even lead to death. Therefore, the strength and conditioning professional needs to be aware of the signs and symptoms of disordered eating and understand who to contact if an athlete is displaying these signs and symptoms.

Anorexia Nervosa
Anorexia nervosa is described as a distorted body image and intense fear of gaining weight. Individuals suffering from anorexia nervosa excessively restrict their caloric intake and are continually worried about their body weight and shape. Furthermore, anorexia nervosa is divided into two subgroups: restricted eating and binge eating or purging. The following provides information on the symptoms associated with anorexia nervosa.

Anorexia nervosa symptoms:

- Brittle hair and nails
- Yellowing skin
- Excessively dry skin
- Fine hair growth over the entire surface of the body, also known as lanugo
- Mild anemia along with muscle wasting and weakness
- Low body temperature
- Constipation
- Hypotension
- Slower breathing patterns
- Bradycardia
- Loss of bone density (osteopenia or osteoporosis)
- Heart arrhythmias or damage
- Amenorrhea and infertility
- Multiple organ failure
- Brain damage

Bulimia Nervosa
Bulimia nervosa is described as a period of considerable overeating followed by a period of purging. Purging can consist of self-induced vomiting, laxative or diuretic use, and excessive exercise. To be considered bulimic, the individual binges and purges at least once a week for a period of three months. Individuals suffering from bulimia nervosa are often more challenging to identify, as their weight is more frequently appropriate for their height. Individuals with bulimia struggle to control their overeating habits but are fearful of weight gain. The following provides information on the symptoms of bulimia nervosa.

Bulimia nervosa symptoms:

- Chronic inflammation of the body
- Sore throat
- Inflamed salivary glands of the neck and jaw

65

- Degeneration or loss of tooth enamel
- Gastrointestinal issues
- Intestinal distress from excessive laxative use
- Severe dehydration from vomiting
- Electrolyte imbalances

Body Composition Changes and Performance Variations Associated With Eating Disorders or Disordered Eating

Although eating disorders are associated with low body weight, this is not always the case. Individuals suffering from anorexia nervosa or bulimia nervosa usually have higher body fat compositions due to the muscle wasting that occurs from such eating disorders. Also, gastrointestinal issues that arise from eating disorders are primarily caused by inflammation, which can lead to excessive gastric emptying. This increase in gastric emptying can lead to further malnutrition and cause the body to lose too many micronutrients. Therefore, the strength and conditioning professional should recognize acute increases in the individual's body fat composition while also monitoring their body weight throughout the training process.

Performance can also be affected by eating disorders, as well as disordered eating patterns. Dehydration, malnutrition, high body fat composition, and muscle wasting can all increase during a time of disordered eating. These side effects tend to increase the potential of injury during exercise. Furthermore, eating disorders can affect the athlete's energy levels. When malnourished, athletes often feel tired and sluggish and fatigue easily. These side effects can be detrimental to performance. Again, any acute changes to energy levels, body compositions, or body weight should be dealt with promptly to address any eating disorder that may be developing.

Referral to a Qualified Health-Care Professional

It is very important for strength and conditioning professionals to understand that they are not responsible for treating individuals who suffer from eating disorders, but they should have the ability to recognize the signs and symptoms of eating disorders and refer the athlete to a qualified healthcare professional. These trained professionals can then develop a treatment program, with a treatment team, to further enhance the effectiveness of accommodating the treatment of the disorder.

Effects, Risks, and Alternatives of Common Performance-Enhancing Substances and Methods

Ergogenic Aids and Dietary Supplements

Strength and conditioning coaches are often approached by athletes who have questions about ergogenic aids that may enhance their performance. Therefore, the strength and conditioning professional should be equipped with knowledge of common ergogenic aids for athletic performance such as creatine, anabolic steroids and their derivatives, and the practices of carbohydrate-loading techniques and blood doping. Some popular ergogenic aids are permitted in sports while others are banned. The strength and conditioning professional should be aware of the potential benefits, side effects, dosage, safety and permissibility of common ergogenic aids that athletes may be interested in.

Creatine

A nitrogenous organic compound, known as *creatine* encourages and helps supply energy to the cells of the human body. Creatine supplementation is very common within the strength and conditioning industry but can also be obtained from natural meat and fish sources. Creatine is primarily stored within the skeletal muscles with a breakdown of approximately 40 percent being in its free form and 60 percent in its phosphorylated form. When creatine is synthesized, it is transported throughout the body via the circulatory system.

During exercise, creatine phosphate or phosphocreatine has a significant role in energy metabolism. Because the amount of ATP stored in skeletal muscle for immediate use can only power a contraction lasting a couple of seconds, the body needs rapid pathways to generate more ATP. Recall that the phosphagen system is the one that can most quickly generate ATP, though the ATP output from the pathway is so small that this system predominantly only powers very short, intense activities lasting ten seconds or less. When a phosphate group is cleaved off ATP (adenosine triphosphate), it becomes ADP (adenosine diphosphate) and energy is released to do work. The ATP is then generated back from the ADP through one of the energy pathways. In the phosphagen pathway, the ADP becomes ATP (which can then supply energy) when phosphocreatine donates a phosphate group to ADP via the enzyme creatine kinase. When phosphocreatine becomes depleted, the ability to perform higher-intensity exercise becomes inhibited. Creatine, either endogenous or from supplementation, can help replace skeletal muscle stores of phosphocreatine, which can be rapidly depleted in high-intensity exercise. Therefore, it can be concluded that most sports that require higher-intensity outputs can benefit from creatine.

Creatine supplementation continues to be one of the most used supplements, especially in collegiate and high school athletics that require high-intensity, anaerobic output. It is estimated that 80 to 90 percent of athletes that compete in a sport that require higher-intensity outputs have supplemented with a form of creatine at some point. Although creatine is widely used, the human body has a finite amount that can be used within a certain time period. Skeletal muscle concentrations of approximately 150 to 160 millimoles per kilogram have shown to be the upper limit in terms of effectiveness during exercise. Once this level is reached, further supplementation will have no benefits to training. Therefore, the mind-set of "more is better" should be substituted for the "minimal effective dose" protocol.

Although creatine supplementation has many benefits, adverse effects can occur. Body mass can increase, which is not always desirable. Increases in body mass seem to be mainly in the form of lean body mass rather than fat, but for sports that require athletes to stay within a certain weight class, the effects of creatine supplementation should be closely monitored. Gastrointestinal issues have also been reported by some users, mainly in the form of digestive distress and diarrhea. Lastly, concerns have risen over the stress placed on the kidneys from creatine supplementation because of the high nitrogen content. However, neither short-term nor long-term creatine supplementation studies have shown any significant dysfunction. That said, the quality of the supplement is important since heavy metals and other undesirable fillers may be present.

Carbohydrate-Loading Techniques

Just as creatine is supplemented to prevent fatigue in strength and power sports, carbohydrate loading is often used in the same manner during long-duration aerobic endurance sports. Carbohydrate-loading techniques are used to enhance muscle glycogen and to prevent the depletion of muscle and liver glycogen, which causes fatigue and a sense of "hitting the wall." Carbohydrate-loading techniques often incorporate a period of loading the body with carbohydrates prior to the onset of activity or competition. Cross-country skiers, road cyclists, long-distance track athletes, and marathoners often use carbohydrate-loading techniques.

Carbohydrate-loading protocols include a three-day loading period, a daily loading period, and a pre-event loading period. The most widely used technique is the three-day loading period. Studies have shown that loading carbohydrates during the three days leading to the athletic event is beneficial for aerobic capacity. This loading period is sometimes preceded by a depletion period where the athlete consciously tries to restrict carbohydrate intake for a few days. Although some studies have shown the three-day loading protocol to be beneficial to both sexes, men seem to benefit more than women. Researchers have concluded this to be based on total caloric intake and the type of carbohydrates used when loading. Glycogen stores do rise in men, but women can have mixed results. When females used carbohydrate-loading techniques in several studies, the daily caloric intake implications seemed to pose a challenge. Women who consumed fewer calories during the period before an event felt sluggish when trying to load carbohydrates in the three days leading to the event. The acute increase, therefore, had little benefit. When administering a carbohydrate-loading period, athletes should consume around 8 to 10 grams per kilogram of body weight during the load phase to enhance muscle glycogen stores. It should be noted that for every gram of glycogen stored, 2.7 grams of water are retained as well, so some athletes can feel heavy and bloated.

Anabolic Steroids
Anabolic steroids are synthetic derivatives of androgen hormones like testosterone that, when used in training and competition, increase testosterone levels, which stimulates protein synthesis. Use of anabolic steroids increases strength, power, and muscular size, which can increase performance in many sports. Many anabolic steroids are created for men with medically-low testosterone levels or wasting diseases like AIDS; the difference between these and those used for sporting purposes is the dosage. Oftentimes, the amount used in athletics is 15 to 20 times greater than that used for medical issues. Furthermore, the use of anabolic steroids is prohibited in most sporting events, professional leagues, and amateur leagues. Sports in which anabolic steroid use is common include strength sports such as football, baseball, powerlifting, and field events in track and field, among others. Also, the use of anabolic steroids has been observed in individuals who do not compete in athletics but who seek appearance benefits. The use of anabolic steroids has shown to increase male characteristics, and using anabolic steroids is more common in men than women, although using anabolic steroids for women is not uncommon.

Throughout training, increases in strength and power are consistently sought. Therefore, one can easily see why using anabolic steroids is prevalent. Within athletic performance, high doses of anabolic steroids contribute to individual athletic success across many different sports. It is important to relay ethical ramifications, as well as risks and detrimental effects, to the athletes, especially within sports with a known history of anabolic steroid use and abuse. Use can also cause high blood pressure, hypercholesterolemia, acne, and liver and kidney disease. Lastly, psychological effects can also be seen with anabolic steroid use, including aggression, arousal, and irritability.

Blood Doping
One of the main limiting factors of success in aerobic endurance events is the body's ability to deliver oxygen-rich blood to the working skeletal muscles. Some endurance athletes turn to blood doping practices to combat this natural limitation. Blood doping can occur from either injecting oxygen-rich blood into the body or by taking a supplement to increase erythropoietin (EPO). EPO stimulates the production of new red blood cells that carry oxygen to skeletal muscle. Although injections and ingesting EPO-stimulating substances are both blood-doping techniques, EPO supplementation has become more common because of its ease of use.

Recombinant human EPO use is developed for patients with anemia or kidney disease to increase their quality of life and is prohibited in most sporting events and competitions. When injections of EPO are administered, increases in both hematocrit and hemoglobin have been observed. Aerobic capacity can be increased by approximately 6 to 8 percent and time to exhaustion can be improved by approximately 17 percent. Therefore, one can easily see the benefits to athletic performance associated with EPO use.

Although EPO is used for patients with kidney disease and anemia, misuse of EPO can have many negative effects and has even been the cause of death in certain occasions. Adverse effects of EPO use include the thickening of blood, hypertension, severe dehydration, and blood clots, strokes, and pulmonary embolisms.

Governing Bodies

Interest from athletes in using performance-enhancing supplements as well as dietary supplements is increasing each year. Therefore, the strength and conditioning professional must be familiar with the major governing bodies of each sport as well as the regulating governing bodies that are used worldwide. Most major sport organizations produce their own list of banned substances and provide useful information that can be accessed by both coaches and athletes. Organizations such as the Major Baseball League, National Football League, National Basketball League, National Hockey League, and the National Collegiate Athletic Association have designated websites to address the banned substances that are prohibited or permitted within their respective sports. Furthermore, national associations such as the World Anti-Doping Agency (WADA), United States Anti-Doping Agency (USADA), and Australian Anti-Doping Agency (ASADA) oversee the doping parameters of the Olympic committees of their respective nation. To ensure athletes consume only safe and effective performance-enhancing supplements, strength and conditioning professionals should familiarize themselves with the common supplements that are often banned by such organizations. Lastly, other valuable resources exist that can further benefit the strength and conditioning professional when determining the legality of supplements. Resources such as Drug Free Sport, Labdoor, and Informed-Choice all have interactive websites that can help determine the usefulness and legality of common performance-enhancing substances and dietary supplements.

Signs and Symptoms of Ergogenic Aid Abuse

Many of the aids used within the strength and conditioning profession pose risks to the body of the consumer. Many of the risks and negative effects are minor with creatine supplementation and carbohydrate-loading protocols. Other ergogenic aids, specifically anabolic steroids, seem to have the more profound negative effects on the human body. Effects from anabolic steroids increase as the dosage increases. These effects include both long-term and short-term risks for the athlete. Therefore, the strength and conditioning professional should attain a thorough understanding of the signs and symptoms associated with ergogenic aid abuse associated with anabolic steroids, particularly because some athletes will not be forthcoming about their use. The following provide some common signs and symptoms of anabolic steroid usage (and some other ergogenic aids as well):

Cardiovascular System
- Hyperlipidemia
- Hypertension
- Myocardial dysfunction

Endocrine System
- Gynecomastia
- Decreased sperm count
- Testicle atrophy
- Impotence
- Increased risk of transient infertility

Male Genitourinary
- Decreased sperm count
- Testicular shrinkage or atrophy

Female Genitourinary
- Amenorrhea or menstrual cycle dysfunction
- Deepening voice
- Clitoromegaly
- Female masculinization

Male and Female Genitourinary
- Changes in libido
- Gynecomastia
- Dermatological issues such as severe, chronic acne on the face and back
- Male pattern baldness

Hepatic
- Increased risk of liver tumors
- Increased risk of liver damage

Musculoskeletal
- Premature closure of the epiphyseal plate
- Abscesses that develop inside the muscle
- Increased risk of tendon tears

Psychological
- Mania
- Depression
- Aggression
- Hostility
- Mood swings

As stated previously, many of the symptoms can be acute and only occur during ergogenic aid abuse, or they can become chronic issues that can take many years to overcome. In either case, many of these symptoms are not conducive to ideal health or performance. Accordingly, such ergogenic aids should not be used by athletes looking to further their athletic career.

Practice Questions

1. In which of the following ways is the cardiovascular system affected by anabolic steroid abuse?
    a. Increased myocardial function
    b. Increased risk in development of liver tumors
    c. Decreased testicular size
    d. Elevated blood pressure

2. Which of the following is the daily protein recommendation for athletes competing in a strength sport?
    a. 1.4 to 1.7 grams of protein per kilogram of body weight
    b. 1.4 to 1.7 grams of protein per pound of body weight
    c. 1.7 to 2.0 grams of protein per kilogram of body weight
    d. 1.7 to 2.0 grams of protein per pound of body weight

3. How many grams of protein should a male American football player consume after a competition?
    a. 10 to 15 grams of protein
    b. 20 to 25 grams of protein
    c. 30 to 35 grams of protein
    d. At least 40 grams of protein

4. Which of the following is a nitrogenous compound that encourages and helps supply energy to the cells?
    a. Branched-chain amino acids
    b. Leucine
    c. Creatine
    d. Nitric oxide

5. What caloric deficit is recommended for the goal of fat loss?
    a. Approximately 250 calories a day
    b. Approximately 500 calories a day
    c. Approximately 750 calories a day
    d. Approximately 1000 calories a day

6. The glycemic index tracks and monitors which of the following physiological responses?
    a. Blood glucose levels two hours after consumption
    b. Blood glucose levels one hour after consumption
    c. Muscle glycogen stores immediately post-exercise
    d. Muscle glycogen stores immediately after consumption

7. Which of the following is a nutritional recommendation for improving muscular endurance?
    a. Low-carbohydrate intake throughout the day
    b. Low-fat intake throughout the day
    c. Protein consumption post-competition
    d. Protein consumption pre-competition

8. Which of the following stimulates red blood cell production?
    a. Calcium
    b. Leucine
    c. Sodium chloride
    d. Erythropoietin

9. Who issued the MyPlate food guidance tool that is commonly used for nutrition information for both athletes and the general population?
    a. United States Department of Agriculture
    b. United States Food and Drug Administration
    c. National Strength and Conditioning Association
    d. National Food and Nutrition Service

10. Which of the following is a symptom of anorexia nervosa?
    a. Smooth, radiant skin
    b. Elevated body temperature
    c. Bradycardia
    d. Hypertension

11. An athlete with a goal of muscle hypertrophy should consume which of the following?
    a. 30 to 100 grams of lower-glycemic carbohydrates post-activity
    b. 30 to 100 grams of higher-glycemic carbohydrates post-activity
    c. 10 to 15 grams of low-leucine protein every two to three hours throughout the day
    d. 10 to 15 grams of high-leucine protein every two to three hours throughout the day

12. Which of the following is NOT considered a psychological effect of anabolic steroid abuse?
    a. Increased aggression
    b. Increased arousal
    c. Increased irritability
    d. Increased relaxation

13. Which of the following is NOT a symptom of disordered eating?
    a. Dehydration
    b. High body fat
    c. Hypertrophy
    d. Muscle wasting

14. How much carbohydrate should be consumed in a pre-competition meal that is consumed at least four hours prior to the athletic event?
    a. 1 to 2 grams per kilogram of body weight
    b. 1 to 4 grams per kilogram of body weight
    c. 4 to 6 grams per kilogram of body weight
    d. 8 to 10 grams per kilogram of body weight

15. Which of the following is NOT a main category of MyPlate recommendations?
    a. Legumes
    b. Fruits
    c. Vegetables
    d. Protein

16. In terms of carbohydrate-loading techniques, which of the following protocols is more popular?
    a. Daily loading period
    b. Pre-event loading period
    c. Week-long loading period
    d. Three-day loading period

17. Which of the following is NOT considered a nutrient-dense food?
    a. Fruits
    b. Banana bread
    c. Vegetables
    d. Lean meat

18. Which of the following is a challenge when attempting to identify an athlete with bulimia nervosa?
    a. They are consistently hydrating.
    b. Their weight loss could be from an increase in energy expenditure and not an eating disorder.
    c. The athlete is often at a healthy weight.
    d. The athlete never consumes food in front of the strength and conditioning professional.

19. Which of the following are the main electrolytes lost in sweat?
    a. Sodium, chloride, potassium, magnesium, calcium
    b. Sodium, chloride, potassium, calcium
    c. Sodium, chloride, potassium, iodine, calcium
    d. Sodium, chloride, potassium, magnesium, iodine

20. Which of the following is considered the limit of creatine storage in the human body?
    a. 40 to 60 millimoles per kilogram
    b. 60 to 80 millimoles per kilogram
    c. 100 to 120 millimoles per kilogram
    d. 150 to 180 millimoles per kilogram

21. Which of the following is NOT a symptom of low iron levels in athletes?
    a. Increased concentration
    b. Increased fatigue
    c. Weakness
    d. Decreased work capacity

Answer Explanations

1. D: Hypertension, or an elevation in blood pressure, is a common side effect of anabolic steroid abuse. The only other answer choice that pertains to the cardiovascular system is increased myocardial function. Anabolic steroids are known not to increase myocardial function but rather to decrease myocardial function.

2. A: For strength sport, it is recommended that athletes consume 1.4 to 1.7 grams of protein per kilogram of body weight daily. This amount is sufficient to sustain muscle protein synthesis and reduce muscle breakdown from training.

3. B: Post-competition nutrition is vital to recovery. Athletes who compete in sports such as American football, which is primarily strength-based and anaerobic, should consume 20 to 25 grams post-competition to reduce muscle soreness and encourage recovery.

4. C: Creatine is a nitrogenous organic compound that helps supply energy to the cells. It is primarily stored within the skeletal muscle of the human body and some is formed endogenously while some is consumed with an omnivorous diet. Supplementation is also common in strength sports and is generally considered safe.

5. B: The recommended daily caloric deficit for safe and effective fat loss is roughly 500 calories per day. This amount will ensure that the body still attains enough calories maintain performance, but the moderate deficit will encourage body fat loss.

6. A: The glycemic index is a ranking system based on how quickly carbohydrates are digested, absorbed, and used as fuel. By using the glycemic index, the athlete can monitor the rate of magnitude of the blood glucose level increase of certain carbohydrate-rich foods in the two-hour post-consumption time period. Food that score lower on the glycemic index are more slowly digested and absorbed than higher-glycemic foods.

7. C: Athletes who are attempting to increase muscular endurance should consume protein post-exercise. This protein consumption will decrease muscle soreness and damage.

8. D: Erythropoietin, or EPO, stimulates the production of new red blood cells, which carry oxygen to skeletal muscle. When injections of EPO are administered either medically or illegally in athletics, increases in both hematocrit and hemoglobin have been observed. This can translate to improved aerobic capacity and endurance.

9. A: MyPlate is a food guidance tool issued by the United States Department of Agriculture that can help athletes understand their basic nutritional needs based on their age, sex, and physical activity. It is important to note that many of the recommendations are based on the needs of the general population rather than those of competitive athletes. However, the recommendations can form a good starting point for a healthy diet for athletes as well.

10. C: It is important for the strength and conditioning professional to recognize symptoms associated with anorexia nervosa. Bradycardia, a slow heart rate, is a common symptom; other symptoms include a decrease in body temperature, hypotension, dull and dry skin, and brittle hair and nails.

11. B: For athletes with a goal of muscle hypertrophy, 30 to 100 grams of higher-glycemic carbohydrates should be consumed after exercise because this will help replenish glycogen stores and encourage protein synthesis. The recommendation for protein is to consume meals that contain at least 20 to 30 grams of high-leucine protein every three to four hours throughout the day.

12. D: Anabolic steroids have many psychological effects on an individual who is abusing the substance. Increases in aggression, arousal, irritability, and mood swings are common. Athletes have also noted the inability to relax when using anabolic steroids.

13. C: Hypertrophy is not a symptom associated with disordered eating. Athletes with disordered eating behaviors often become malnourished, which makes hypertrophy impossible. Furthermore, dehydration, higher body fat composition, and muscle wasting have all been associated with disordered eating patterns.

14. B: For meals that are consumed four or more hours prior to the athletic endeavor, athletes should consume 1 to 4 grams of carbohydrates per kilogram of body weight in a balanced meal containing protein and healthy fats. Hydration is also important.

15. A: MyPlate is a great starting point for athletes to evaluate their current diet and should be used to identify areas within the diet that are lacking. MyPlate categorizes foods into five main components: fruits, vegetables, grains, protein, and dairy. Legumes, although often consumed by athletes, are not a main component of MyPlate. They can provide a good source of protein, especially for vegetarians, and complex carbohydrates.

16. D: The most widely used carbohydrate-loading technique is the three-day loading period protocol. Studies have shown that this timeframe helps increase endurance during aerobic exercise such as marathon running.

17. B: Nutrient-dense foods are foods that have many micronutrients, vitamins, and minerals along with their macronutrients of carbohydrates, fats, and protein. Banana bread is not considered a nutrient-dense food but rather a calorie-dense food.

18. C: Individuals suffering from bulimia nervosa are often more difficult to identify, as they are more frequently at a normal weight for their height. The binging behavior can prevent weight loss, even when accompanied by purging behaviors.

19. A: Electrolytes lost in sweat need to be replaced to prevent imbalances and deficiencies. The main ones to consider are sodium and chloride, though potassium, magnesium, and calcium are also excreted in sweat and need to be replaced. Iodine is not lost in appreciable levels during exercise.

20. D: Although creatine is widely used, the human body has limits on how much can be used during a certain time period. Skeletal muscle concentrations of approximately 150 to 180 millimoles per kilogram have shown to be the upper limit of the effective concentration during exercise. Once this level is reached, further supplementation will have not benefit performance.

21. A: Low iron levels occur in three different stages of increasing severity: depletion, marginal deficiency, and anemia. When anemia is prolonged, red blood production ceases, which reduces oxygen transport throughout the body. Low iron levels can cause difficulty concentrating, fatigue, weakness, decreased exercise and work capacity, and dry mouth.

Exercise Technique

Proficiency in exercise technique is vitally important for the strength and conditioning professional. Understanding the movement patterns and helpful verbal cues for each exercise not only provides a safe and effective training environment but can also decrease the likelihood of injuries. Fortunately, many exercises used within the strength and conditioning profession have similar body position and instructing techniques for one exercise, can often help the athlete perfect his or her technique on other exercises as well. Understanding the commonalties within movement patterns will help simplify the complex movement systems of the human body.

Resistance Training Exercise Technique

Free Weight Training Equipment

Preparatory Body and Limb Positioning
Free weight training equipment usually involves the use of barbells or dumbbells for external resistance. Whenever the body has an external load placed upon it, the athlete must start with a stable and rigid position. This position may vary slightly depending on whether the athlete is lying on the floor or bench (supine position) or standing erect before executing the movement. In either case, the body must be stable to maintain proper spinal alignment while allowing the limbs to move fluidly. This stable position often starts with the Valsalva maneuver while the spine is in a natural, neutral position.

The Valsalva maneuver involves inhaling using deep belly breathing and then increasing abdominal pressure by trying to exhale while holding the glottis closed. This built-up abdominal pressure helps maintain a neutral spine, which increases the stability and safety of the movement or exercise.

Many occasions may call for use of a weightlifting belt. Weight belts have the ability, when used correctly, to augment the pressure induced by the Valsalva maneuver by increasing abdominal pressure and further enhancing spinal stability. It is important for the strength and conditioning professional to teach athletes when and how to use weight belts properly while training. Weight belts should be used during movements that place a high load on the spine and during maximal efforts. When movements are not stressing the spine nor attempting maximal percentages, the use of a weight belt is not warranted and may be contraindicated because it reduces the muscular involvement of the core.

When the athlete is performing exercises on a bench (whether flat, decline, or incline) or if the athlete is lying supine on the floor), a five-point position must be achieved to ensure the body is stable against the bench or floor. The strength and conditioning professional can explain this position by starting from the athlete's feet and moving toward the head. The first two points of contact of the five-point position are the feet. Both the right foot and left foot must be flat on the ground, and pressure must be applied through the foot to ensure that the foot does not move during the exercise. The third point of contact for support is the glutes, which will be in contact, and stay in contact, with the bench or floor during the entire execution of the exercise. Fourth, the upper back, from thoracic spine to cervical spine, will also stay in contact with the bench or floor during the entire exercise. Lastly, the back of the head will be in contact with the bench or floor.

Grip position plays a vital role in attainment of proper technique in nearly every exercise and can vary greatly depending on the goal of the movement. There are many different grips, and it is important to understand each type. The pronated grip, or overhand grip, is the most common grip when using a barbell or dumbbell. The pronated grip is the position when athletes look at their hands and see the back of the hand where the knuckles are. The supinated grip is the opposite of the pronated grip. In the supinated, or underhand grip, the palms are facing up, and the knuckles and back of the hand are facing downward. The neutral grip is different than the previous two in that the palms are facing each other, and when looking at the hands, the thumb and the index finger are visible to the athlete. Lastly, the alternated grip is usually shoulder-width apart with one hand in the pronated grip position and the other hand in the supinated grip position. This grip is usually necessary in near-maximal deadlift attempts but should be used with caution, as it can alter the stability of the exercise when it is used as a primary grip position. When the athlete is performing Olympic lifts, two different grips are used: the clean grip and the snatch grip. As the name implies, the clean grip is used for the clean and its variations. It involves the hands positioned slightly wider than shoulder-width and is often a comfortable racking position for the catch of the clean and the front squat. The snatch grip is wider than the clean grip and is usually close to or outside the power rings on an Olympic barbell. This grip is used for the snatch and its variations and the catching position in the snatch and overhead squat.

The final step in preparing the athlete for free weight exercises is grip width and stance. The appropriate grip width depends primarily on the goal of the exercise and can vary widely among different movements. When looking at a standard Olympic barbell, three different types of grip widths will be used: narrow, common, and wide. The narrow grip requires the athlete to place his or her hands closer within the knurling of the barbell. The common grip width requires hands to be shoulder-width apart, usually between the start of the knurling of the barbell extending to the first power ring (the non-knurled ring break between knurling sections). The wide grip width extends beyond this power ring on an Olympic barbell.

Stance follows the same principles as grip width in that it is determined based on the goals of the movement, but the common stance for standing exercises is a comfortable shoulder-width stance with the toes pointed slightly out to ensure the knees are tracking appropriately and not putting any excessive pressure on the hip, knee, or ankle joints (essentially, this is the athletic stance position). A common verbal cue given to the athlete is to have them prepare to take a vertical jump, and before leaping, look down at the feet. This positioning of the feet usually puts the athlete in the correct stance for most free weight exercises done in an erect position.

With an understanding of stability, grip width, and stance, the athlete is now prepared to start movement. Throughout the movement, these factors must be maintained to execute the exercise safely and effectively.

Execution of Technique

In free weight training, it is important to understand the basic, fundamental movements of the body. With this understanding, the strength and conditioning professional will be able to promptly correct any issues that may arise during the execution of the exercise. Any exercise that places stress on the lower limbs will require a specific position of the upper body to protect the spine from any harm during the movement. As the athlete is already in an athletic position, it is important for them to attain a chest-up position, shoulder blades pulled back with downward pressure to ensure they do not move, a flat back (neutral spine), and the head looking straight ahead.

The Athletic Position

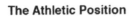

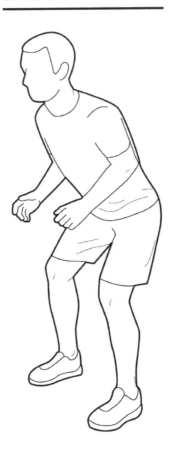

In many instances, the athlete will look upward or downward during the execution of the exercise. This position may place excessive stress on the spine because it forces the spine out of its normal anatomical position. When the athlete is performing exercises for the upper body, the feet will stay stationary on the floor, and pressure will be placed on the feet and lower limbs to prevent them from moving. Next, as the exercise is performed, the athlete must be aware of the breathing patterns during the movement. During every exercise, there is a portion of the movement where the force will peak. This portion of the movement is termed the *sticking point* of the exercise, and the athlete should learn to exhale during this time. The athlete will then inhale during the portion of the exercise when the external force is lower. It is common to inhale during the eccentric portion of the exercise, perform the Valsalva maneuver during the change of direction portion of the exercise, and exhale during the sticking point.

It is also important for the athlete to focus on certain aspects of each exercise. When attention is placed on critical components of each exercise, the athlete will be less likely to focus on irrelevant stimuli that could cause inefficient or incorrect movements. It is advantageous to have the athlete go through certain focal points during the exercise. Using a set routine for points of focus helps the athlete ensure that the movement is performed in a safe manner. Taking the squat as an example, the athlete could have the following routine for focal points: chest up, back flat, chin neutral, breath into abdomen, control the eccentric phase, push through the heels, and power on the concentric phase. Therefore, each area of the movement will have a specific focus, and the exercise will be more productive.

Another area the strength and conditioning professional must be familiar with is the athlete's mental state. Each athlete will be slightly different in the level of excitement necessary for optimal conditions on free weight training, and it is important to get to know each athlete on an individual basis. Once the strength and conditioning professional gets to know the athlete, any major differences in day-to-day training can be identified. The athlete's state of mind can have major implications on the outcome of the exercises for that day, and it will be very dependent on the intensity of the exercise. For example, sets of three repetitions at 90% intensity will require the athlete to be "locked in" in terms of focus, and the arousal of the athlete should be optimal. In another situation, the athlete may not need the same intensity of arousal for sets of three repetitions at 70% intensity of the same exercise. If the athlete were to have the same arousal levels in both situations, the arousal state may be too constant, and the body will not have the same response when greater levels of arousal are needed for higher workloads.

Correction of Improper Technique

If and when the strength and conditioning professional witnesses an athlete using improper technique, it is important to correct the issue immediately. If the improper technique is not corrected at that moment, the incorrect movement pattern will start becoming engrained into the athlete's movement pattern. In such an instance, communication is the key to success. The ability to communicate effectively during the training process is a bit of an art, and it is important for the strength and conditioning professional to consistently work on this skill.

As stated many times before, when utilizing free weights, especially when the barbell is placed on the back for lower-limb exercises, it is important to ensure the spine is in a neutral position. During the execution of the exercise, it is common for the upper back to lose some lose stability, and the back may round. As many free-weight exercises place a bar on the athlete's back, it is important to understand how to correct this fault. By cueing the athlete to keep their chest up during the movement, the stability and rigidness of the spine will tend to correct itself. Another fault that is common with lower-limb free-weight exercises is for the knees to track inward instead of tracking out, but not beyond, the toes. The main reason for this inward tracking of the knees is due to strength imbalances in adductors and abductors. To correct this common issue, verbally cueing athletes to keep an outward pressure on the lower limbs as they move through the exercise will usually correct the technical flaw. When the use of a bench or floor is warranted, as in upper-limb horizontal movements, focus should be on stabilizing the core while the upper-body limbs are moving. If any of the five points (left foot, right foot, glutes, upper back, and head) lose contact with the contact points, a prompt correction should be made to ensure the body stays stable and rigid. Many improper technique issues arise when the athlete is not taught proper form or when the weight of the barbell increases too rapidly. To correct this issue, it is important to take ample time to teach the athlete the exercises and to advance them in an appropriate manner to ensure proper adaptations are made during the training process

Resistance Machines

Resistance machines are exercise units that utilize a cam, a pulley, hydraulics, air resistance, or lever-based external resistance to the body. Unlike multi-joint free-weight exercises, resistance machines primarily stress one or two body parts at a time. Resistance machines are not only a common modality for strength training, but they are often used for rehabilitation. Because the athlete is usually placed within an exercise machine that is then adjusted for the individual, resistance machines are usually less complicated than free weights.

Preparatory Body and Limb Positioning

It is important to have a basic understanding of each individual resistance machine that will be utilized during the training process. Having this understanding will give the strength and conditioning professional the expertise needed to ensure the resistance machines are used in a safe and effective environment. Many of the resistance machines have moving parts that can be adjusted for each individual's limb lengths and anthropometry. Each resistance machine operates around an axis that places external resistance on the primary muscle group and joint targeted by that machine. It is important to place the athlete so that his or her body is stable and appropriate stress is applied to the working muscle groups. Once the machine is adjusted and the athlete is in a proper, stable position, the exercise can be executed. It is important to note that adjustments may need to be made between sets or repetitions as the joint angles change.

Execution of Technique

When using resistance machines that place stress on the lower limbs of the body, the athlete's hands will be placed on the handles of the machine to stabilize his or her body. When the machine targets the upper body, the lower limbs or feet will either be placed into pads or held stable against the ground. Depending on the machine's axis of movement, these stability points may change, but it is important to have at least one stable body point to ensure maximal force can be developed by the body. As resistance machines primarily use single-joint movements, it is imperative that a full range of motion is used. When the athlete, or the resistance machine, limits the range of motion, an excessive amount of stress can be transferred to the joints of the body. When range of motion is limited, often more weight can be used but the athlete is not performing the exercise correctly, which can cause injury and certainly reduce the effectiveness of the exercise. Therefore, it is important for the athlete to utilize the full range of motion while executing any exercise on a resistance machine. As the athlete is executing the movements when using resistance machines, control is of major concern. Anytime the athlete uses uncontrolled movements, the risk of injury is high and the machine can also be damaged. Each segment of the exercise may require a different pace of movement so that the athlete can remain in control and perform the exercise safely. Often, when using resistance machines, there will be a point when the primary mover undergoes its peak contraction. Having the athlete "squeeze" or flex the muscle maximally during this peak portion of the exercise can enhance the effectiveness of the movement.

Correction of Improper Technique

Common corrections that the strength and conditioning professional must be aware of are proper alignment before executing the exercise, maintaining stability during the movement, ensuring that the body stays in contact with the pads during execution, using an appropriate pace for repetitions, and controlling each movement. With awareness of these points, the strength and conditioning professional can ensure a safe, efficient, and effective training environment while utilizing resistance machines.

Alternative Modes

In certain situations, a strength and conditioning professional may utilize alternative modes of strength training, depending on the purpose of training. These alternative modes consist of body weight exercises, core, stability, balance, and calisthenics. The advantage of alternative modes of training is that there is very little equipment needed to successfully perform the training, which can take place in areas that typical free weights and resistance machines are not usually seen (e.g., outdoors and in open gymnasiums). These training methods may be warranted as precursors to other types of training, as the amount of external resistance is less than that of other modes.

Preparatory Body and Limb Positioning

Preparing the body for alternative modes is very similar to preparing for free-weight training. There may be times when more emphasis is placed on the attainment of proper stability, as many of the core, stability, and balance methods may put the athlete in an unstable environment. Therefore, it is important to teach proper mechanics, such maintaining a neutral spine, keeping the chest up, and the chin in the neutral position. As many modes of alternative training have athletes using their own body weight for resistance, it is also important to teach them to keep the elbows in before performing upper body exercises to ensure the athlete is not putting too much external rotation onto the shoulder region. Once the athlete has a basic understanding of the proper body-positioning cues of alternative modes, they can begin movement of the body.

Execution of Technique

Whether athletes are performing body-weight, core stability, unstable environment, or balance training exercises, they should be under control during the entire execution of the movement. Focus and attention are vitally important to ensure that the body stays under control. Athletes should be focused on the task at hand while also monitoring their center of gravity as their body is moving through space. By placing the focus and attention on the body and not on external stimuli, he or she will be less likely to lose stability and balance throughout the exercise. When body weight exercises are performed, it is important to note that there will not be any other aspect to focus on besides the body itself. Because of this, these exercises can serve as a good first starting point to master before doing weighted exercise because the athlete will develop a base of understanding about how his or her body performs under such movements. As athletes moves through the movement of any alternative mode of training, their posture should remain neutral throughout the entire movement. If at any time the athlete starts to round his or her back, the chest starts to cave inward, or the chin deviates from its natural position, immediate attention should be placed on correcting the issue. This can be a great method for learning the athlete's weaknesses and identifying specific positions where the athlete losses stability.

Training with bands and chains also falls within alternative modes of training. These are balance exercises, as the use of bands and chains will change the trajectory of the barbell if stability and balance are lost during the execution of the movement. The use of bands or chains is termed "accommodating resistance," and it is important for the strength and conditioning professional to understand the use of this method of training. Throughout movement, especially with multi-joint free-weight exercises, there will be portions of the movement that are less stressful to the body due to different angles of the joints. During these portions of the movement, bands or chains can be used. Bands and chains are placed on the barbell and, when properly applied, can increase the stress on the body during the less intensive portions of the movement. When using these types of alternative training methods, it is important to understand that the stress on the body is greater, making them more stressful to the central nervous system.

Correction of Improper Technique

As the use of alternative methods of training primarily places the body in environments where forces change throughout movement, it is vital that the strength and conditioning professional communicate clearly with the athlete during the entire movement. Many times, necessary corrections are to enhance or fix proper body alignment throughout the exercise. If at any time the body is not in a correct position, direct focus should be placed on correct alignment during that portion of the exercise. Having ample time to instruct the athlete is important when utilizing alternative methods of training. Too often the athlete will be rushed through this acclimation period and proper mechanics will not be developed.

Non-Traditional Implement Training

The use of logs, tires, weighted push sleds, sand bags, stones, and kettlebells is known as non-traditional implement training. This type of training has become more popular in recent years and is a new way to add external resistance to the body. Many times, the use of non-traditional implements will place the athlete in unstable environments, along the same lines of alternative training methods, which increases the demand on core musculature and the real-life sports application of the movement.

Preparatory Body and Limb Positioning
Whenever a non-traditional implement is lifted from the ground, proper body alignment is needed. Ensuring that the back is flat, the chest is up, and the chin is neutral is important in preparing the athlete to lift these implements from the ground, especially if the implement will be lifted from the ground and walked or run to a different position. When using tires for training, it is important for the athlete to be taught the proper movement mechanics, as they are different than any other style of training. When flipping a tire, the upper body can be placed onto the tire, increasing the stability of the body against the non-traditional implement. To increase the stability of the body against a tire, the athlete should learn to lean against the tire while performing the Valsalva maneuver. Attaining this stability will place a tremendous amount of stress onto the upper core of the body, increasing the effectiveness of the movement. When preparing the athlete to lift or throw an object overhead, it is important for them to set up so the implement will not come in contact with anything other than the hands of the athlete. Some modifications may be warranted to ensure there is a clean path for the implement.

Execution of Technique
The specific type of non-traditional implement being used will have great implications on the execution of the exercise. That said, it is important that the body stays in a proper position throughout the movement and that stability is always maintained throughout the exercise. As with many other modes of training, the athlete should always maintain a neutral body position that is conducive to the training implement. One main teaching point, when using non-traditional implements, is to ensure the athlete is using their entire body to lift the implement and that the entire body is working in succession. The hips, knees, and ankles should all be working together when lifting non-traditional implements. If, at any time, the athlete only uses one of these three joints when lifting an object from the ground, a segment of the body will endure more stress than it should, making the movement unsafe.

Correction of Improper Technique
To ensure the athlete is lifting the non-traditional objects with proper technique, the strength and conditioning professional must be aware of the requirements for the lift to be successful. Placing the feet too close together can put too much load on the spine and the knees. Placing the feet too far apart can put too much load onto the hips and lumbar spine. It is also important to ensure that the implements are moved in a smooth, controlled manner. Whenever the athlete jerks to lift the object, the hips will rise too quickly and a high load will be placed on the back. Ensuring that the hips and shoulders rise together is important. Also, whenever the athlete loses stability during the execution of the movement, he or she should be taught the proper way to release the movement to ensure that the implement does not come back down onto the body, potentially injuring the athlete.

Plyometric Exercise Technique

Plyometric exercise consists of movements that place an emphasis on the stretch-shortening cycle of both muscles and tendons and usually involve explosive movements. Using plyometric training, athletes will increase their power development by means of training peak maximal force in the shortest time. In terms of athletic performance, the athlete who can produce the most force or attenuate force rapidly and accelerate in an opposite direction will have an advantage over his or her competition. Therefore, the use of plyometric training exercises can become vitally important for the strength and conditioning professional to implement in an athlete's training program. In any plyometric exercises, there will be a loading on the muscles of the body. This loading period will occur during the eccentric (lowering) portion of the movement. Once the energy is loaded into the muscles and tendons, there will be a brief period when the body changes direction. This period is termed the *amortization portion* of the exercise, and is when the muscle contraction shifts from eccentric to concentric. Once the brief amortization period occurs, the muscles generate force through concentrically. The eccentric, amortization, and concentric periods make up the main components of any plyometric exercise. For plyometrics, both lower- and upper-body exercises can be performed. Lower-body plyometric exercises include box jumps, depth jumps, multiple hops and jumps, standing jumps, skips, jumps in place, and bounds. Upper-body plyometric exercises include bilateral medicine-ball throws, unilateral medicine-ball throws, catches, and many dynamic pushup variations.

Preparatory Body and Limb Positioning

Before executing any type of lower-body plyometric exercise, it is important to teach the athlete how to properly set up for a jump, both bilaterally and unilaterally, and how to land. For most lower-body jumps, the shoulders should be aligned over the knees and midfoot. Ensuring that all three (shoulders, knees, midfoot) are aligned is important in attaining the proper starting position for lower-body plyometric exercises. When using pushup variations for upper-body plyometric exercises, the athlete should maintain a neutral spine at all times. As plyometric exercises place high forces on the body, especially upon landing, the neutral spine position is challenging, but critical, to maintain. Shoulder and elbow positioning is also important. When more force is placed on the upper body, such as in plyometric upper-body exercises, the elbows will tend to point more anterior than is optimal. This is mainly due to the body trying to compensate for the force applied to the upper body. When preparing athletes, it is important to ensure they keep the elbows closer to the torso, allowing the shoulder to stay in anatomical position. Before executing the exercise, the athlete should be stable in the proper starting position, with the core held tight, the back in its neutral position, and head looking forward.

Execution of Technique

When performing lower-body plyometric exercises, whether vertical or horizontal, it is important to begin with a slight countermovement. This countermovement will have the athlete back on their heels, allowing all lower-body posterior chain muscles to engage. By engaging the posterior, lower-body muscles, the body will be able to apply more force by using the stretch-shortening cycle. The stretch-shortening cycle will lead to the amortization phase of the exercise. Again, this portion of the exercise is very brief, and force will be generated at maximal levels. After the amortization phase, the athlete will shift their weight from the heels to the toes and generate force concentrically, producing the main movement of the exercise. During the eccentric portion of the movement, the lower-body joints will flex slightly. After the slight flexion of these joints and during the concentric portion of the movement, the hips, knees, and ankles extend. During the concentric phase when all joints are extending, it is important to achieve total hip, knee, and ankle triple extension in maximal range of motion. Without achieving full extension in any of the lower-body joints, force production will be inhibited, and the exercise will not be that effective.

When utilizing vertical plyometric lower-body exercises, it is important that the force is applied in an upward movement and that the body is prevented from moving forward or backward during the execution of the exercise. Whether performing single or multiple jumps, it is important for the athlete to land with proper mechanics. One area of concern is the knees. When landing, the knees should flex and stay in a constant angle from each other to best absorb body weight. A helpful cue the strength and conditioning professional can provide is to have the knees pushed out when performing and landing the jump. If the athlete is consistently showing signs of the knees caving in upon landing, strengthening exercises should be given to strengthen the abductors to increase the stability of the knee.

While performing lower-body plyometric exercises, the arms will move as well. During the countermovement of the exercise, the arms will swing down and back to apply move force to the lower body, increasing the strength of the stretch-shortening cycle. During the amortization phase, the arms will become weightless as they start to move upward during the concentric action of the movement. It is important for the athlete to use the arm movement with power, as this will increase the efficiency of the exercise and make the movement more successful. When doing multiple hops and jumps, it is imperative that the athlete attempts to decrease the ground contact time with maximal effort. The more time spent on the ground in multiple jump exercises, the less effective the stretch-shortening cycle will become.

Upper-body plyometric exercises that use of medicine balls can produce great forces for many athletes. To execute these types of exercises, the athlete will begin in a stable position. When standing, the athlete should be in an athletic position with the core and spine in a stable position and head looking forward. If supine, the athlete should have a five-point position on the floor and the core stable. As with lower-body plyometric exercises, the upper-body movements begin with a countermovement. This movement requires the athlete to cock his or her arms back toward the torso, generating power via the stretch-shortening cycle. Using proper arm action, the athlete then throws the medicine ball by punching through the air while keeping the elbows tucked into the side. When throwing a medicine ball overhead or toward the ground, the elbows should stay locked in as the countermovement produces force through the upper back and serratus anterior muscles. Many medicine ball exercises involve two athletes working together. It is important for the training partners to be sufficiently far apart to ensure the velocity of the medicine ball decreases before it reaches the partner. If the partners are too close, injury from the force of the medicine ball can occur.

Pushup variations can also be used for upper-body plyometric exercises. When utilizing pushup variations in this manner, it is important that the body stays stable. The shoulders and knees should remain in a straight line, ensuring there is no flexion or extension at the torso. The countermovement begins when the athlete eccentrically lowers the body to the ground or a medicine ball. After the amortization and during the concentric portion of the movement, maximal force should be applied as the body begins ascending away from the floor.

Breathing is important during any plyometric exercise. The ability to maintain stability during the movements is highly dependent on the ability to hold a stable breath during the amortization phase and through the beginning of the concentric portion of the exercise. The body will attain a natural style of breathing during these phases, and only faulty breathing patterns should be corrected.

Since plyometric exercises use such a high intensity for the enhancement of the athlete, arousal levels should be high when attempting such movements. If the athlete approaches the exercise in a low arousal state, the exercise will not be performed at a high enough intensity to induce positive training adaptations. Ensuring that the athlete is in the correct state of mind before any plyometric program is imperative to the success of the program.

Correction of Improper Technique

Athletes should constantly be monitored throughout plyometric exercises to ensure proper biomechanics are used; otherwise, improper technique needs to be corrected. An increase in knee stress due to a valgus knee angle can pose a significant injury risk to the athlete. When knee valgus is observed, it is imperative to ensure the athlete is made aware of the issue and that correction to proper movement mechanics happens promptly. If the knee valgus continues, the strength and conditioning professional must regress the plyometric program and use less-intensive modes for power production. The use of a box may become necessary, as less force is applied to the knee when jumping onto a surface compared to the stress encountered when landing freely. Another common correction is that of lumbar hyperextension. When the athlete loses stability of the spine and torso, it is common for the power produced to transfer to the lower spine and cause hyperextension. If the athlete were then to land in a hyperextended position, injury may occur. To correct this issue, the strength and conditioning professional must ensure that a stable spine is always maintained throughout the entire movement, including the landing position. While instability is less common in upper-body movements, it can be seen in some pushup variations. Often this instability will occur when the athlete nears his or her limit in terms of volume (repetitions and sets), wherein the athlete may no longer be able to hold a stable position in the concentric phase of the pushup. To correct this issue, the strength and conditioning professional must look at the programing of the training session and adjust the volume of the upper body plyometric portion of the program.

Speed/Sprint Technique

Strength and conditioning professionals must understand the basic biomechanical and physiological aspects of sprinting mechanics and be able to teach athletes how to attain these positions during training. Speed and sprint training can make a major impact on the training program but must be programmed to ensure that proper recovery is given during intense bouts of sprint training, which can have a major impact on the central nervous system.

Preparatory Body and Limb Positioning

Before beginning the sprint training session, the athlete must first understand the basic fundamentals of sprinting. To assist this, the strength and conditioning professional must slow down the movements so the athlete can learn the proper limb position in each phase of sprinting and follow the instruction. The athlete's elbows should flex to around 90 degrees, with the hands in a comfortable, natural, static position. The static hand position should not be too tight nor too loose. The athlete's chest should stay up and out so the shoulders are able to move in a natural, unbroken rhythm throughout the sprint. The core should remain stable without any excessive rotation from side to side while the hips move naturally. During the strides, the lead leg flexes as the back leg extends while pushing through the ground. The knee of the lead leg flexes to the point where the gastrocnemius muscle and ankle become close to the posterior thigh. Throughout the sprinting motion, the ankle will cycle through dorsiflexion and plantarflexion. Again, it is important to slow down these movements when first teaching the athlete to aid comprehension.

Execution of Technique

Sprinting can be broken down into phases: the start phase, the acceleration phase, and maximal velocity. When starting, the athlete should either be in an upright position, in a downward position in a three- or four-point stance, or in a downward position in starting blocks. When the athlete is in any of the downward positions, the lead leg should be flexed around 90 degrees and the trailing leg should be flexed to around 130 degrees. When starting, the athlete should focus on applying maximum force through the ground with both feet to propel his or her body forward horizontally. Within the first couple of strides, the athlete transfers the force from horizontal displacement to gradual vertical displacement. As the athlete runs, the arms work together to have an opposite arm/opposite leg action. This arm action is usually natural, but it is important that the athlete focus on utilizing the full range of motion, especially when starting from a static position.

As the body starts to rise in the first couple of strides, the top of the lead legs will start to rise from a perpendicular position to a more parallel position relative to the ground. The athlete's arms move through a position where the hand is close to the hip and the elbow is pointed straight back to one where the hand moves up towards the face with the elbow pointed ahead. Ensuring that the elbows are staying close to the body is important so rotational forces aren't decreasing the force applied into the ground. When the lead leg is in flexion, the ankle should be in dorsiflexion. When that same leg contacts the ground in the early-support phase, the ankle will start to transfer from dorsiflexion to plantarflexion throughout the support series. The force will transfer all the way through the heel to the toes and begin the flight series.

There are four segments that explain each motion of the lower legs throughout the sprinting movement. The first segment is the *eccentric braking period* of the lead leg. Here, the lead leg is extended, the ankle is pointed toward the knee, and the knee is slightly flexed to ensure that it does not lock out terminally. Once the transfer is made through the foot, the next segment, called the *concentric propulsive phase*, begins. During this time, the lead leg applies a vertical force to the ground to propel the body forward. As this segment occurs, the lead leg is pulled under the body until it releases from the ground. As the athlete propels, the lead leg becomes the trailing leg as it reaches the next segment known as the *recovery phase*. During the recovery phase, the ankle starts dorsiflexing and the knee starts flexing as it recovers and prepares for another ground contact. *Ground preparation* is the last segment. As the trailing leg starts to prepare to become the lead leg, the knee flexes to the same position that it acquired during the eccentric braking segment. Throughout these segments, the head and neck will remain in a neutral position, looking straight ahead.

Sprint Mechanics

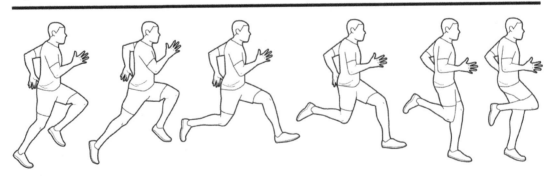

Correction of Improper Technique

It is important for the strength and conditioning professional to slow down the sprint mechanics when analyzing sprint movements. By slowing down the movements, the athlete will begin to feel each movement segment as the body propels forward. Video analysis can also be helpful since the athlete can still sprint at maximal speed but the review can be slowed down as much as necessary. Once proper mechanics are established, the athlete can start to increase the intensity of the movement. As the intensity is increased, it is important that the athlete does not lose form on any phase or regress to previously-established poor mechanics. Some scenarios may require the athlete to remove certain sprint movements to focus on other aspects. An example would be having the athlete kneel as they progress through arm action drills focusing on proper arm placement as the intensity increases. Sprint mechanic work can be thought of as a constant progression and regression, as improper movement patterns present themselves.

Agility Technique

Much like speed, agility can play a vital role in athletic preparation of the athlete. Agility is the ability to accelerate, decelerate, and rapidly change direction and make precise movements. Understanding proper movement mechanics is very important for the strength and conditioning professional.

Preparatory Body and Limb Positioning

The athlete will begin by attaining a basic athletic stance with the ability to move forwards, backwards, and laterally. This position will have the athlete aligned so the feet are close to shoulder-width apart, the chest is held high over the toes, the knees ae slightly flexed, and the posterior chain muscles are engaged. Once in this position, the athlete should focus on the stimulus to which he or she will react.

Execution of Technique

Now that the athlete is in the proper position, he or she will be able to react to the training stimulus used in the given drill. The execution of the movement will begin by extending the hips, knees, and ankles, regardless of the direction. The athlete should be focused on pushing through the ground with maximal force to fully accelerate the body in the proper direction. In many agility drills, the athlete must decelerate and reaccelerate in an opposite direction. To begin the deceleration process, the torso should remain neutral; too much lean of the upper body must be prevented. If the athlete leans too much into a turn, more force is required to regain balance. As the athlete is decelerating, the hips should flex, allowing the center of gravity to move lower as the chest maintains its position over the midfoot. During both acceleration and deceleration movements, the legs and arms should work together. Focusing on powerful arm actions in proper directions will increase the force produced by the lower limbs, which increases the efficacy of the drills. As the athlete is moving through the drills, focus should be placed on the reactive stimulus used. If another athlete is used, focus should be placed on this other athlete's shoulders, torso, and hips. As agility drills are reactive in natural, maximal intensity is often needed for the drill to be successful. Arousal levels should be high, and the athlete's focus should be honed on the external stimulus.

Correction of Improper Technique

As the athlete is moving through the drills, attention must be placed on flexing the hips, knees, and ankles upon deceleration. Often, athletes can be observed changing direction with a stiff, extended leg. This can be very unsafe, as it places high forces on the joints of the body. To prevent this, the strength and conditioning professional should allow adequate time to progress the athlete through proper movement mechanics. Other common improper techniques include leaning too far when changing direction, keeping the head in an unnatural position, and moving the legs and arms in quick, choppy actions. To correct these issues, the strength and conditioning professional may need to regress the athlete to slower drills to reinforce proper movement.

Metabolic Conditioning and Energy System Development

Strength and conditioning professionals need to understand the metabolic demands on the athlete for his or her given sport to best help prepare the athlete to perform at a high level and recover well for the next session.

Cardiovascular Equipment

When utilizing cardiovascular equipment for the attainment of metabolic conditioning and energy system development, it is important to have a basic understanding of the equipment. Designing workouts involving treadmills, stair steppers, stationary bikes, rowing machines, and elliptical strength and conditioning professionals are common in the strength and conditioning profession, and understanding how to properly use each machine will benefit the strength and conditioning professional in terms of knowing how when, and why to incorporate these modalities into an athlete's program.

Machine Programming and Setup
Treadmill
The treadmill can be used in many different scenarios. The use of a treadmill is often warranted, whether the goal is to have the athlete increase circulation and mobility prior to a workout, correct improper running or walking gait, develop the cardiovascular system, keep the athlete safe during bad weather, or improving certain energy systems. When utilizing a treadmill, the athlete will begin by placing the safety switch attachment to his or her body. The safety switch attachment should be placed so it does not contact any moving limbs, as this can pull the cord and cause the treadmill to shut off inadvertently. Once the safety switch attachment is placed onto the body and the safety key is inserted into the treadmill, the athlete will stand straddling the belt of the treadmill. The speed, incline, or specific program can now be set according to the goals of the training session. Once these are adjusted, the athlete will begin by allowing one foot to step onto the belt to attain a perspective on the speed and prepare the body for the speed of the movement. Once the body is prepared, the athlete can start fully utilizing the treadmill. Whether walking, jogging, or running, it is important that the athlete stays toward the front of the belt, ensuring they do not fall off the back when fully striding. Throughout the movement, the athlete should stay tall in nature and keep the eyes looking forward to maintain balance while moving. Natural running gate should be mandated throughout the entire training session. Unless specifically indicated for some reason, the athlete should not hold onto the side railings. Normal arm movement should accompany locomotion on the treadmill.

Bicycle
Many times, especially when low-impact exercise is desired, the use of a stationary bicycle is warranted. The strength and conditioning professional will begin by having the athlete sit in an upright position on the seat of the bicycle. From here, adjustments to the height of the seat are made so the athlete's extended leg is still slightly bent at the bottom portion of pedal rotation. Terminal knee extension is to be avoided during the downward pedal stroke; at least five or ten degrees of knee flexion should occur. Once the seat position is adjusted, the height of the handlebars can also be adjusted to ensure the athlete is in an upright position and the shoulders are prevented from rounding forward while pedaling. The midfoot should stay in contact with the pedals of the bicycle throughout the pedal stroke. The athlete will begin by slowly building up the rotation speed of the pedals while maintaining an upright position throughout the training session. Once the workout is complete, the athlete will begin to slow down the speed of the pedals until the they come to a complete stop.

Rowing Machine

The rowing machine is an excellent modality when whole-body conditioning exercise is needed. To begin, the athlete will sit on the pad of the machine and attain an upright position while keeping the shoulders back and the head looking forward. The athlete will extend the arms and hold onto the rowing handle while flexing the hips and knees and maintaining a neutral spine. To start the exercise, the athlete will extend the knees and hips from the flexed position and pull the rowing handle towards the torso. To increase or decrease the intensity of the exercise, adjustments to the air vent can be made to increase or restrict air flow into the console of the rowing machine. Once the knees and hips are fully extended, the elbows flexed, and handle is near the torso, the recovery phase can occur. The recovery phase starts by flexing the knees and hips, and then arms, as the body comes closer to the machine's console.

Stair Stepper

The stair stepper is another example of a low-impact conditioning tool often used in the strength and conditioning industry. The athlete will begin by placing the hands onto the handrails and placing each foot onto the respective foot pedals. Once aligned on the machine, the intensity or program can be selected. Once ready, the athlete will begin by flexing one knee and allowing the pedal to retract upwards. When the pedal retracts around four to eight inches, a downward pressure will be applied as the opposite pedal comes upward in the same manner as the previous pedal. During movement, the body will stay upright in a natural position, the knees aligned over the toes, the toes pointed forward, and the hips aligned with the torso. During movement, the toes should continue to face forward, and this alignment should be maintained during the duration of the training session.

Elliptical Strength and conditioning professional

The elliptical strength and conditioning professional is a good modality when higher intensity and lower impact is needed. The athlete will begin by placing the feet on the respective pedals. The hands will grasp the upright handlebars. The athlete will begin the movement by moving the arms and legs together as if running or jogging. The lower limbs will reciprocate with the machine in a natural fashion. It is important that the athlete maintain a natural proper position with the chest held high, back flat, head looking forward, and shoulders relaxed.

Preparatory Body and Limb Positioning

When utilizing cardiovascular equipment for metabolic conditioning and energy-system development, there are certain guidelines that must be maintained throughout the exercises. First, it is important that the body stays in a natural position throughout the entire training session. Often during fatigue, the shoulders will round, and the athlete will start to hunch over. Maintaining a natural body position ensures the exercise will be performed in a safe and effective manner. During the use of each piece of equipment, the back must maintain a neutral spine, the chest should stay tall, head looking forward, and shoulders relaxed. By maintaining this posture, the lungs will be able to perform work at the highest capacity, making the exercise more effective.

Execution of Technique

While utilizing cardiovascular equipment, it is important that the athlete uses a natural gait throughout each exercise. This gait will be individualized and therefore adjustments may need to be made to the equipment. The strength and conditioning professional should also note the athlete's breathing when using cardiovascular equipment. Breathing should be natural and controlled throughout the exercise, especially when reaching higher intensities. The athlete may need to be taught proper breathing mechanics when utilizing cardiovascular equipment to enhance the effectiveness of the exercises. Focus and arousal levels for the athlete will depend on the intensities used for each training session. For example, a lower-intensity training session will require less focus and arousal from the athlete than a higher-intensity session where higher heart-rate levels are to be achieved. Knowing how the athlete responds to different cardiovascular stimuli can greatly affect the outcome of the training session.

Correction of Improper Technique

Many of the corrections that will need to be made during cardiovascular equipment training sessions will be that of positioning and posture. Positioning on the machines becomes vitally important in ensuring that the athlete is in proper body alignment in relationship to the machine. Posture cues must be given when fatigue starts setting in and the athlete starts having a difficult time maintaining proper position, especially during higher-intensity training sessions. Ensuring that the athlete is in the proper position in relationship to the machine and maintains proper alignment throughout the training session will greatly enhance the effectiveness of the equipment.

General Body-Only Activities

In many occasions, cardiovascular equipment may not be available, and the strength and conditioning professional must have the athlete engage in body-only activities for metabolic conditioning and energy-system development. These activities may include walking, jogging, running, and swimming. It is important to understand proper mechanics when using such activities during the training process.

Execution of Technique

Whether walking, jogging, or running, the athlete will be in an upright position with the aligned with the torso, the shoulders relaxed, and the head upright, while the eyes are focused ahead of the athlete. During movement, the heel of the athlete contacts the ground first. Once heel strike occurs, pressure moves from the heel toward the midfoot in a rolling fashion. Pressure should also be placed on the outside of the bottom of the foot to maintain the natural foot arch. During the activity, the hips extend and flex during the natural stride as the athlete propels forward.

Arm action is also important to note during walking, jogging, and running exercises. As the right leg is coming forward, the left arm should be coming forward. As the left leg is coming forward, the right arm should be coming forward. Natural movement at the shoulder is needed when utilizing these types of exercises. Throughout arm action, the elbow should stay flexed around 90 degrees and the hands should be in a relaxed position. The hands should come as high as the chest or sternum during upward motion and back to the lateral hip in the downward motion.

Breathing considerations must be made when utilizing body-only activities. For less-intensive training, the athlete will maintain a natural breathing pattern. When training intensities are higher, more attention must be made to maintain this pattern. For the athlete, attention and focus should remain on proper mechanics during the training session.

Correction of Improper Technique

Faulty movement mechanics, especially in repetitive conditioning activities, increases the likelihood of injuries. Therefore, it is important to establish an effective line of communication so the athlete can be informed when faulty movement mechanics appear.

Anaerobic Conditioning Activities

Anaerobic training can be very beneficial to the athlete, especially when training for athletic performance. The amount of conditioning drills and modalities used for anaerobic training is endless. Understanding basic movement will help the strength and conditioning professional when utilizing anaerobic training.

Execution of Technique

Many forms of anaerobic training involve sprinting. While the goal of this type of training is to induce positive adaptations, it is important to note that these types of exercises can be very demanding on the athlete, and the need for proper movement mechanics is paramount to reduce the risk of injury and induce the desired benefits. For drills involving running, the athlete should perform all activities while keeping his or her chest up, back flat, chin neutral, and shoulders relaxed. The same movement patterns hold true for activities in which bodyweight exercises are used intermittently. Maintenance of a stable athletic position is the correct execution for many intermittent training sessions.

Breathing will be natural throughout the anaerobic training sessions, although more rest time may be warranted if the athlete shows improper breathing patterns. Focus and attention for the athlete should be shifted towards proper positioning at the task or modality of the training session. As many anaerobic training sessions are intensity-driven, arousal levels should be high. The higher-intensity sessions will require the athlete to be focused and alert during each portion of the intervals and ready to perform each exercise at the maximal intensity.

Correction of Improper Technique

Proper positioning is a concern when administering any type of anaerobic training, especially when intermittent intervals are prescribed. The strength and conditioning professional should make sure to have a clear line of communication with the athlete to ensure any faulty movement patterns can be corrected. If at any time faulty movement patterns are seen, the strength and conditioning professional should stop the activity and possibly regress to a lower-intensity exercise until proper conditioning and strength are attained.

Flexibility Exercise Technique

Static Stretching Exercises

The utilization of static stretching can improve range of motion, enhance recovery, or form a component of an injury rehabilitation program. As such, static stretching has proven to be a beneficial tool for the strength and conditioning professional.

Preparatory Body and Limb Position

Knowledge of muscle attachments (regarding origin and insertion) will help the strength and conditioning professional select the appropriate stretches for an athlete and instruct the positions correctly. Before performing any type of stretching, it is important for the athlete to perform a general warmup to move blood from the organs to the muscles, increase the body's core temperature, and prepare to attain an effective range of motion during the stretching. When performing static stretching, the athlete's body should be relaxed. Once the body is relaxed, the athlete should take a deep breath into the abdomen, control the breath, and exhale into the stretch.

Execution of Technique

Once the athlete is in proper position and the body is relaxed, he or she can begin by slowly reaching through the beginning range of motion. The entire movement should be controlled, without any jerking motions. As the athlete increases the range of motion at the joint, normal breathing should occur so the body stays relaxed throughout the entire movement. Once the athlete attains a range of motion where there is mild discomfort, movement should stop, and the athlete should hold that position for 15 to 30 seconds. If the athlete is doing a unilateral static stretch, the stretch should be performed on both sides of the body to facilitate full-body stretching. Arousal and focus are important factors when utilizing static stretching exercises. Arousal levels should be low to allow the body to relax and attain a full range of motion for the exercises. When performing static stretching exercises, the athlete should be focused on the muscles that are stretching and should strive to attain the full range of motion to increase the effectiveness of the exercise.

Correction of Improper Technique

For correction of improper technique to occur, the strength and conditioning professional must be familiar with proper stretching mechanics. Most corrections will come from faulty movement patterns and the inability to become relaxed while experiencing the mild discomfort that results from static stretching. Relaxation techniques may be needed to facilitate achieving full range of motion in the exercises. If at any time during the 15-second hold body position starts to change, the strength and conditioning professional must instruct the athlete to maintain proper position. The tendency to move out of proper position is common if the athlete is new to static stretching or unfamiliar with the exercise.

Proprioceptive Neuromuscular Facilitation

Proprioceptive Neuromuscular Facilitation, or PNF, involves the strength and conditioning professional assisting in stretching exercises while utilizing contractions at different positions to inhibit and relax tight or tense muscles. The role of the strength and conditioning professional in PNF stretching is to instruct when contractions are to occur and to provide external resistance onto the athlete's body.

Preparatory Body and Limb Positioning

After a general warmup that increases blood flow, heart rate, and core temperature, the athlete should align themselves in a natural, relaxed position and the strength and conditioning professional should align themselves in a position where they can apply external resistance onto the muscles being stretched. Once each participant is in their respective positions, the stretching exercise can begin.

Execution of Technique

During PNF stretching, three techniques can be used: the hold-relax technique, the contract-relax technique, and the hold-relax technique with agonist contraction. Each position will be explained using a PNF hamstring stretch as an example.

The Basic Hamstring Partner Stretch Position

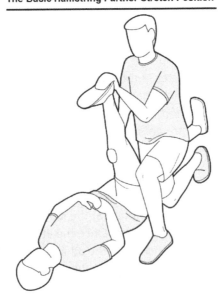

When utilizing the hold-relax technique, the movement begins in a basic supine hamstring stretch where the athlete is in the point in the range of motion where mild discomfort is felt. This first basic stretch should last for 30 seconds. The strength and conditioning professional should have one hand placed on the athlete's knee and the other on the heel to maintain stability of the lower limb. The strength and conditioning professional should instruct the athlete to hold this position and prevent the strength and conditioning professional from moving the limb as the strength and conditioning professional applies pressure to the limb. This pressure is applied for six seconds. After six seconds, the athlete will relax, and another static-partner stretch will occur for another 30 seconds. The second stretch during the relaxation phase should attain a greater range of motion than the previous stretch.

The contract-relax technique also begins in a basic supine hamstring stretch, and the athlete will attain the point in the range of motion where mild discomfort occurs. This beginning stretch will be held for 10 seconds. The athlete will apply pressure to the external resistance provided by the strength and conditioning professional and contract his or her hamstring by extending the hips. This contraction will occur during full hip extension in a normal range of motion. Once the entire range of motion is attained, the athlete will relax, and the second-partner stretch will occur. The second-partner hamstring stretch will occur for 30 seconds and should attain a greater range of motion than the previous stretch.

The hold-relax with agonist contraction will start by using the hold-relax technique for the first two portions of the exercise. The only change in this technique is the final phase. During the final phase, the athlete will contract the agonist muscle of the exercise, increasing the total range of motion for the movement. This greater range of motion is due to reciprocal inhibition, the hips activating during flexion, and autogenic inhibition during hamstring activation.

Correction of Improper Technique

While most techniques during PNF stretching should be closely monitored, it is also important to clearly communicate during each phase of each movement. If, at any time, the athlete feels too much pressure, he or she must communicate with the strength and conditioning professional to ensure injury does not occur. Communication is also key during certain phases when the athlete must contract or hold during the exercises.

Dynamic Stretching Exercises

Dynamic stretching exercises occur when the athlete is performing stretching exercises through active movement. A greater range of motion is usually achieved during dynamic exercises than during static exercises.

Preparatory Body and Limb Positioning

The athlete should prepare for movement in a relaxed, natural position. The athlete's eyes and head should be focused ahead and his or her breathing pattern should be normal. Before dynamic exercises, the athlete should have performed a general warmup to increase core temperature and joint elasticity.

Execution of Technique

When performing dynamic stretching exercises, the athlete should start with a smooth and controlled repetition and progress slowly, increasing the range of motion on each repetition. The athlete should perform 5 to 10 repetitions of each exercise, whether performing the exercise in place or throughout a given distance. If having the athlete perform the exercises for a distance, it is important that the distance relates to the amount of space needed for each set. As the athlete moves through a series of exercises, ensure that he or she is only moving at the targeted joint. Any other movement will result in faulty movement patterns where the body is compensating for some inflexibility.

Correction of Improper Technique

If the athlete starts the exercise in a rapid movement, injury may occur from compensating body parts. To ensure the movement is performed in a controlled manner, the strength and conditioning professional should have the athlete progressively move through the joint's full range of motion. Any bouncing movement (a faulty movement pattern) should be addressed and the athlete should control his or her body through the entire exercise.

Spotting Procedures and Techniques

One of the main roles of a strength and conditioning professional is to implement training exercises to the athlete that are safe and effective. As safety is the most important goal in strength and conditioning, the use of a spotter is needed on any exercise that places the external load over the athlete's head, on the back, anteriorly on the clavicles, or over the face. The only exception is during power exercises. Power exercises do not require a spotter, as the athlete should be properly trained to successfully abort the exercise when the weight becomes unmanageable.

Number of Spotters Needed for a Given Situation or Exercise

Exercises that warrant the use of one spotter:

- Bench press
- Incline dumbbell bench press
- Flat dumbbell fly
- Forward step lunge
- Step-ups
- Seated barbell shoulder press
- Lying barbell triceps extension

Exercises that warrant the use of two spotters:

- Back squat
- Front squat

Spotter Location

It is important to understand the location of the spotter to prevent an unsafe training environment and maintain the balance of any external resistance when assistance is needed. Clear communication and focus is just as important for the spotter as it is for the athlete. For exercises that utilize one spotter, the spotter should be located either behind the athlete (forward step lunge, step-up, and seated barbell shoulder press) or above the athlete's head for supine lying exercises (bench press, incline dumbbell bench press, flat dumbbell fly, and lying barbell triceps extension). For exercises that utilize two spotters, each spotter should be positioned to the side of the barbell within reach to assist the athlete if needed.

Body and Limb Placement Required When Spotting the Lifter

Body and limb placement depends on the exercises. For exercises that require the athlete to be lying in a supine position, such as the bench press, incline dumbbell bench press, flat dumbbell fly, and lying barbell triceps extension, the spotter should stand anterior of the athlete's head with his or her feet about shoulder-width apart and a with slight knee flexion. Although proximity to the athlete is needed, the spotter should never be in the athlete's line of sight during execution of the exercise. For horizontal

94

pressing movements, any time the athlete needs assistance when beginning the lift (lift-off), the spotter should hold the barbell with an alternated grip inside the grip width of the athlete. Although the spotter's hands are on the barbell at lift-off, they should be removed once the exercise begins. During execution of the exercise, the spotter should keep his or her hands near the barbell or dumbbell, but unless assistance is needed, the spotter should not touch the barbell or dumbbell. During the concentric portion of the movement, the spotter should extend his or her knees to attain a higher position and move along with the ascending barbell or dumbbell. If dumbbells are used, the spotter should contact the athlete's wrist instead of the dumbbells so that balance is maintained throughout the movement.

During lower body movements that require the use of one spotter (forward step lunge and step-up), the spotter should be behind the athlete with his or her feet around shoulder-width apart and the knees slightly flexed. As the athlete begins the movement, the spotter should step forward, with the same leg as the athlete, and keep his or her hands near the athlete's hips and torso. As the athlete performs the concentric phase of the movement, the spotter should move in unison so that contact is not made with the athlete, unless assistance is needed. With all these exercises, the spotter should always assist the athlete in racking the barbell or setting down the dumbbells.

When performing the back squat and front squat, the use of two spotters is needed. When performing these exercises, the spotters should stand in an erect position at opposite ends of the barbell and maintain slight knee flexion. To assist in un-racking the barbell, the spotters should hold onto the bar and walk back, in unison, with the athlete. Once the athlete is balanced, the spotters should release the barbell but keep their hands in proximity to the barbell in case assistance is needed. As the athlete begins the eccentric portion of the movement, the spotters should flex their knees and move along the same path as the barbell. In the concentric phase, the spotters should extend their knees, keeping their chests tall, and move in unison with the athlete. Once the set is completed, the spotters should grasp the bar and assist in racking the barbell onto the squat stands or rack.

Practice Questions

1. During multiple hops or jumps in plyometric training, what should that athlete focus on during the time spent in contact with the ground?
    a. Increase ground contact time to ensure full force is applied on every jump
    b. Allow the body to naturally absorb the pressure of the body upon landing
    c. Keep the legs extended to increase the braking technique
    d. Reduce ground contact time to ensure a fast rate of force development

2. Which of the following is NOT a correct body position when using a stair stepper machine?
    a. Knees aligned over the toes
    b. Toes pointed forward
    c. Head looking upward
    d. Spine in a neutral position

3. Which of the following is a technique used to increase resistance during the portion of the exercise where typically there is less resistance?
    a. Accommodating resistance
    b. Force-velocity technique
    c. Manual resistance
    d. Intensity increase technique

4. During speed and sprint training, which of the following techniques can be used to improve the athlete's movement patterns?
    a. Having the athlete perform each movement as quickly as possible to improve technique at high speeds
    b. Slowing down the movement of the drill to attain proper mechanics before increasing intensity
    c. Providing verbal training cues while the athlete moves through the full intensity speed drill
    d. Performing technique work while using upper and lower limbs consecutively

5. During the front squat, where should the spotters be located?
    a. In front of the athlete
    b. Laterally, to each side of the barbell
    c. Behind the athlete with their hands placed on the barbell
    d. Spotter are not needed for the front squat

6. What is the muscle action of the hip during the midflight phase of a sprint?
    a. Concentric flexion
    b. Eccentric flexion
    c. Concentric extension
    d. Eccentric extension

7. Where are the hands located while utilizing a narrow grip width on an Olympic barbell?
    a. Near the center of the barbell, where there is no knurling
    b. On the knurling, outside the first power rings
    c. Near the center of the barbell while still in full contact with the knurling
    d. A thumbs-distance away from the smooth part of the barbell

8. When utilizing resistance machines for training, which of the following will NOT increase the effectiveness of the exercise?
    a. Making sure the athlete's body stays in contact with the pads
    b. Making the tempo of the movement as explosive and powerful as possible
    c. Achieving full range of motion on every repetition
    d. Making sure the athlete utilizes the Valsalva maneuver while executing the exercise

9. What is the purpose of the slight countermovement that occurs when doing plyometric exercises?
    a. To use more momentum when executing the exercise
    b. To apply more force by actively engaging the stretch-shortening cycle
    c. To engage the entire musculature of the body
    d. To increase pressure placed on the joints

10. When fatigued, which of the following is a common fault observed during conditioning exercises?
    a. Shoulders start to round forward
    b. Spine starts to hyperextend
    c. Relaxed breathing patterns
    d. Head starts to lean back

11. During agility drills, which of the following describes the position of the hips upon deceleration?
    a. The hips stay extended and the center of gravity is high
    b. The hips rotate in the direction of the movement
    c. The hips stay static and do not move
    d. The hips will flex as the center of gravity becomes lower

12. During free weight resistance training, which of the following positions should be maintained to ensure a safe and effective exercise?
    a. Back flat, chest rounded, and head looking upward
    b. Back in hyperextension, chest up, and the head looking downward
    c. Back flat, chest up, and head in a neutral position
    d. Back flat, chest up, and head looking upward

13. The five-point position for the bench press includes which of the following?
    a. Left foot on floor, right foot on floor, glutes on bench, upper back on bench, back of head on bench
    b. Left hand on barbell, right hand on barbell, head on bench, upper back on bench, glutes on bench
    c. Left foot on bench, right foot on bench, left hand on barbell, right hand on barbell, back on bench
    d. Left foot on floor, right foot on floor, glutes on bench, upper back on bench, back of head tucked and off the bench

14. For lower-body plyometric exercises, which of the following ensures the athlete's body is in proper alignment?
    a. The chest is rounded, knees are located over the ankles, and the athlete's weight is shifted to the heels
    b. The head is anterior to the knees, the hips are located back, and the athlete's weight is shifted towards the toes
    c. The spine is hyperextended, knees pointed slightly towards each other, head is looking straight ahead
    d. The shoulders, knees, and mid-feet are in line with each other when looking at the athlete from the side

15. On a treadmill, what must occur before the machine will turn on?
    a. The safety switch must be inserted, and the attachment must be placed on the athlete's body
    b. The machine must be wiped clean
    c. The treadmill must be set at a slight incline
    d. The athlete needs to start with a warmup

16. Which of the following accurately describes agility?
    a. Acceleration through changes in direction
    b. The ability to accelerate, decelerate, and rapidly change direction
    c. The ability to decelerate and hold the body stable in a static position
    d. The ability to maintain balance in unstable environments

17. While training at 85% intensity for a set of 5 repetitions, the athlete's focus and arousal should be at which of the following levels?
    a. Focus high, arousal low
    b. Focus high, arousal high
    c. Focus low, arousal low
    d. Focus low, arousal high

18. When should the strength and conditioning professional make corrections to faulty movement mechanics that occur during the training process?
    a. The next training session when the athlete is fully rested
    b. After the set of repetitions is performed
    c. Promptly, even if it interrupts the training set or repetitions
    d. It is not needed, as the athlete will feel the faulty movement and correct it themselves

19. When would the use of a weightlifting belt be warranted?
    a. While the athlete is performing warmup sets
    b. During exercises that place a low load on the spine
    c. While attempting percentages that require maximal effort
    d. While using upper-body resistance machines

20. When flipping a tire, where should the chest be placed to increase the athlete's stability?
    a. Away from the tire, using the Valsalva maneuver
    b. Against the tire, using the Valsalva maneuver
    c. Rounded away from the tire
    d. The chest is not a main concern when flipping a tire

21. Where should the knees be placed upon landing during lower-body plyometric exercises?
    a. In a staggered stance to actively dissipate the load of the body
    b. Together, to increase joint stability at the ankle
    c. Outward, to ensure maintain a constant angle relative to each other
    d. Fully extended, to prevent the body from absorbing too much pressure

22. When administering exercises that require the athlete to run, jog, or walk, where should the pressure on the foot be located to ensure the natural curvature of foot arch?
    a. Towards the heel
    b. Towards the ball of the foot
    c. Towards the medial portion of the foot
    d. Towards the outside of the foot

23. Which of the following does NOT require the use of a spotter?
    a. Bench press
    b. Back squat
    c. Lying barbell triceps extension
    d. Power clean

24. Which of the following is NOT a technique used for proprioceptive neuromuscular facilitation?
    a. Hold-relax technique
    b. Relax-release technique
    c. Contract-relax technique
    d. Hold-relax technique with agonist contraction

25. Where should the athlete's hands be located when using a lower-body resistance machine?
    a. Clasped together, on the back of the head
    b. Grasped firmly on the handles of the machine
    c. Crossed across the athlete's chest
    d. Feeling the lower-body muscles contracting

26. Which of the following accurately describes the pronated grip used for the barbell Romanian deadlift?
    a. While looking down, one hand will be facing palm up while the other is palm down
    b. While looking down, both hands will be facing down, with knuckles up, in an overhand grip
    c. While looking down, both hands will be facing upright, with knuckles down, in an underhand grip
    d. While looking down, the palms will be facing one another, and the knuckles will be outward

27. When high force is placed on the athlete during upper-body plyometric exercises, what is a common mistake made by the athlete during the execution of the exercise?
    a. The head lifts off the ground when pushing forward
    b. The feet move away from the body as the power is generated for the exercise
    c. The elbows flare out and more pressure is added to the shoulder girdle
    d. The hips move forward as the athlete attempts to produce maximal power for the movement

28. When performing cardiovascular exercise on a rowing machine, how does the athlete or strength and conditioning professional increase or decrease the resistance of the machine?
    a. Adjust resistance on the seat of the machine
    b. Adjust the air vents to allow or restrict air flow
    c. Adjust resistance on the rowing handle of the machine
    d. Adjust the console of the machine

29. Which of the following occurs during a general warmup?
    a. Core temperature increases
    b. Muscles tighten
    c. Central nervous system fatigues
    d. Range of motion decreases

30. What is the term used for the portion of the movement where the force of the external resistance will peak due to joint angles?
    a. Peak point
    b. Maximal force zone
    c. Full-intensity position
    d. Sticking point

31. Which of the following accurately describes the amortization phase during plyometric training?
    a. The eccentric, lowering action of the body before the concentric muscle action
    b. The concentric, upward movement of the body
    c. The counteraction of the body to increase the stretch reflex
    d. The phase between eccentric and concentric muscle action of the body

32. When adjusting a stationary bicycle to the needs of the athlete, what position should the knee be in at the full downward stroke of the pedal?
    a. The knee should be terminally extended
    b. The knee should be in flexion around 90 degrees
    c. The knee should be flexed 5-10 degrees
    d. The knee should be slightly extended

33. What can be done to ensure proper breathing patterns are maintained during anaerobic conditioning?
    a. Intensities can be increased
    b. Rest periods can be decreased
    c. Water can be given to the athlete
    d. Rest periods can be increased

34. All EXCEPT which of the following are benefits of static stretching?
    a. Increased range of motion
    b. Enhanced recovery
    c. General body warmup
    d. Useful as a corrective exercise

35. If the athlete is continuously showing signs of the knees caving in during hip, knee, and ankle free-weight exercises, which of the following would NOT be a good verbal command for the technical flaw that needs correcting?
    a. "Keep outside pressure on the way up."
    b. "Keep your hips engaged throughout the movement."
    c. "Keep your chest up during the entire movement."
    d. "Your knees should track over, but not beyond, the toes.'

36. Which of the following is NOT a segment of lower-limb breakdown of sprinting mechanics?
    a. Eccentric braking period
    b. Concentric propulsive phase
    c. Ground preparation phase
    d. Acceleration phase

37. What is the placement of the hands relative to the body when utilizing proper arm action during running, walking, and jogging?
    a. During the upward movement, the hand should reach the as high as the chest and during the downward movement, the hand should reach as low as the lateral hip
    b. During the upward movement, the hand should reach as high as eye level, and during the downward movement, the hand should reach as low as the naval
    c. During the upward movement, the hand should reach as high as the jaw, and during the downward movement, the hand should as far back as the glutes
    d. During the upward movement, the hand should reach the as high as the chest, and during the downward movement, the hand should reach as low as the anterior hip

38. During the first couple of strides of a sprint, how does the force displacement shift?
    a. From horizontal displacement to vertical displacement
    b. From vertical displacement to horizontal displacement
    c. From transverse displacement to vertical displacement
    d. From transverse displacement to horizontal displacement

Answer Explanations

1. D: Reducing contact time should be the athlete's goal during multiple hops and jumps in plyometric training. During plyometric training, putting attention and focus on the reduction of ground contact time will reduce the amount of time spent on the ground, increase the rate of force development, increase power, and increase the ability of the body to utilize the stretch-shortening cycle.

2. C: If the athlete were to keep his or her head in an upward position, too much load would be placed on the cervical spine while it was in an unnatural curvature. With an unnatural curvature of the spine, breathing mechanics can become inhibited, decreasing the effectiveness of the metabolic conditioning.

3. A: Accommodating resistance is the technique of using bands or chains in training to increase the force throughout portions of the exercise where resistance is less. While training, attention may be placed on the force-velocity curve of certain exercises. It is important for the strength and conditioning professional to understand different modalities available for the attainment of enhanced performance.

4. B: By slowing down the movement of the drill, strength and conditioning professionals will be able to make the proper adjustments to the athlete's sprint mechanics before increasing the intensity of the run. If the athlete were to perform drills at maximum speed without making corrections to improper technique, it is more likely that improper movement patterns would become further engrained. Technique proficiency should be mastered at lower intensities and slower speeds before performing drills at higher intensities.

5. B: Placing spotters on each end of the barbell ensures a safe environment when performing the front squat exercise. Any other position of a spotter would unbalance the barbell in cases where assistance is needed. If the strength and conditioning professional were to stand in front of the athlete, focus and attention may be lost during the exercise. Furthermore, because the barbell is anterior relative to the athlete, a spotter in the posterior position would not offer enough assistance.

6. A: During midflight, the hip will concentrically contract and flex as it prepares for ground contact. This concentric muscle action of the hip will prepare the athlete for another stride as the opposite leg is beginning to become uncontacted with the ground.

7. C: In the narrow grip, the hands grasp the barbell close to one another while still utilizing the knurling of the barbell. By placing the hands closer together, no knurling would be available and the exercise would not be performed in a safe environment. If, at any time, the knurling is not used, the barbell could slip out of the athlete's hand causing harm or injury.

8. B: While utilizing resistance machines for the attainment of performance enhancement, the tempo, or rate, of the movement should be controlled and performed in one fluid motion. Performing the exercise in a fast and explosive manner would put an excessive amount of stress on the athlete, especially in the eccentric phase of the exercise. Instead, the strength and conditioning professional must ensure that the movement is performed in a controlled manner while the athlete maintains full contact with the pads of the machine. Also, the use of a full range of motion and performing the Valsalva maneuver will increase the effectiveness of the movement.

9. B: By utilizing the stretch-shortening cycle, the athlete will increase force development by engaging the proprioceptors in the muscle bellies and tendons, which can signal the brain to increase force production in the effector muscles. The countermovement, when used in plyometric training, will actively engage muscles that would not be activated if the countermovement were not performed.

10. A: When the athlete becomes fatigued during conditioning exercises, the shoulders tend to start to round forward. This position can decrease the effectiveness of the aerobic system (because the chest cavity, diaphragm, and lungs can be compressed. This can place strain on the tissues and decrease the intake of oxygen. The strength and conditioning professional must ensure proper body alignment is maintained throughout the entire duration of the exercise.

11. D: As the athlete decelerates, the hips should flex, allowing the center of gravity to drop lower as the chest maintains its position over the midfoot. With a lower center of gravity, the athlete will be able to apply maximal force when beginning to accelerate. If the athlete were to keep the hips extended and the center of gravity high, he or she may become unbalanced, and more time would be needed to attain proper position for changing direction.

12. C: By maintaining a flat back, chest up, and neutral head position, the athlete will be performing free-weight exercises in a safe and effective manner. If the back were to round or hyperextend, too much stress could be placed on the spine, and injury could occur. The chest-up position will assist the athlete in maintaining stability throughout the movement and the neutral position of the head will ensure the athlete is not placing too much load on the cervical spine during the movement.

13. A: It is important that the strength and conditioning professional ensures the athlete is stable throughout the entire execution of the barbell bench press. To maintain stability, the five-point position must be employed. First, the right foot must be flat on the ground and pressure must be applied through the foot to ensure that it does not move during the exercise. The second position is that of left foot being in the same position of the right one. The glutes form the third point of contact. The should be in contact with the bench or floor during the entire execution of the exercise. Fourth, the upper back from thoracic spine to cervical spine must stay in contact with the bench or floor during the entire exercise. Lastly, the back of the head, by the occiput, should be in contact with the bench or floor.

14. D: Proper body alignment is critical in plyometric exercises. Any exercise that is performed when the body is not properly aligned will cause improper movement mechanics and place a tremendous amount of stress on the athlete's body. Keeping the shoulders, knees, and mid-feet in line with each other during the movement can ensure that proper body alignment is maintained throughout the exercise. Whether the athlete is performing the countermovement, the concentric extension portion, or the eccentric landing portion of the exercise, it is important to ensure that this body position is maintained for safety.

15. A: Any treadmill used during training should be properly equipped with a safety switch. A treadmill without a safety switch is a safety concern and should not be used. By having working knowledge of a treadmill, the strength and conditioning professional will be properly prepared to conduct safe sessions.

16. B: Agility is defined as the ability to accelerate, decelerate, and rapidly change direction. Although acceleration through changes in direction, the ability to decelerate and hold the body in a static position, and the ability to maintain balance in unstable environments are all components of agility, in isolation, they do not describe agility.

17. B: When training at 85% intensity, five repetitions would be considered a maximal-effort repetition range. Therefore, the athlete's focus and arousal levels should both be high. If the focus and arousal levels were lower immediately preceding and during the exercise, it is unlikely that the athlete would have a successful attempt in performing all five repetitions. It is important for the strength and conditioning professional to understand what intensities warrant higher and lower arousal levels and mentally prepare the athlete for the programmed intensities.

18. C: During exercise, faulty movement patterns may occur. It is important that the strength and conditioning professional identify and correct these patterns promptly to prevent such errors from further engraining themselves in the athlete's mind. If the strength and conditioning professional were to wait or not correct the faulty movement pattern, athletes could injury themselves. Less critically, the athlete's performance may also fail to reach its potential.

19. C: Many occasions call for use of a weightlifting belt. Weight belts have the ability, when used correctly, to increase the effectiveness of the Valsalva maneuver by increasing abdominal pressure. This will further enhance the stability of the spine. It is important for the strength and conditioning professional to teach athletes when and how to properly use weight belts while training. Weight belts should be used for movements that place a high load on the spine and during maximal weight training efforts. When movements are not stressing the spine or are at submaximal efforts, the use of a weight belt is not warranted. If the athlete were to use a weightlifting belt on every exercise, proper core strength could be inhibited, and the athlete could start to rely too much on the weightlifting belt.

20. B: Tires have become very popular in non-traditional implement training, and proper technique is vital in ensure they are used in a safe manner. When using tires for training, it is important for the athlete to be taught the proper movement mechanics because they are different than any other style of training. When flipping a tire, the upper body can be placed onto the tire, increasing the stability of the body. To increase the stability of the body against a tire, the athlete should learn to lean against the tire while performing the Valsalva maneuver. This will increase the safety and effectiveness of the movement.

21. C: As relative loads can be very high during lower-body plyometric training exercises, it is important to ensure the knees are properly absorbing the loads of the body upon landing. When landing, the knees should flex in parallel, absorbing the weight of the body in a healthy joint angle. A common cue to give is to have the knees pushed out when performing and landing the jump. If the athlete's knees are caving in upon landing, strengthening exercises should be given increase the stability of the knee. Failing to do so can increase the likelihood of knee injuries, especially to the ACL.

22. D: To ensure proper heel strike, pressure should be placed toward the outside of the foot. By placing the pressure on the outside of the foot, the natural arch will be maintained throughout the exercise and the load will be appropriately dispersed. If the arch becomes flattened through excessive repetitions, biomechanical issues can arise from improper balance and loading from the hips, knees, and ankles.

23. D: While most exercises will require the use of a spotter, it would be very difficult and unsafe to attempt and spot a power clean due to the force and velocity applied to the barbell. The other choices (bench press, back squat, and lying barbell triceps extension) must use a spotter. Although the power clean does not warrant the use of a spotter, it is important to teach the athlete to properly abort the exercise if technique ever becomes faulty.

24. B: The three techniques used for proprioceptive neuromuscular facilitation are the hold-relax technique, the contract-relax technique, and the hold-relax technique with agonist contraction. As PNF stretching is widely used in the strength and conditioning profession, it is important to have a thorough understanding of the terminology and techniques used with PNF stretching.

25. B: While utilizing resistance machines during training, it is important to attain and maintain stability throughout the entire movement. During the use of lower-body resistance machines, the athlete's hands should be placed firmly on the handles of the machine. Any other hand placement could cause the athlete to become unbalanced and unstable when executing the exercise.

26. B: Having a thorough understanding of proper hand placement is advantageous for strength and conditioning professionals and their athletes. A pronated grip is widely used on many exercises in the strength and conditioning profession. The pronated grip is the most common grip when using a barbell or dumbbell. The pronated grip occurs when the athlete looks at their hands and sees the back of the hand where the knuckles are.

27. C: Shoulder and elbow positioning is important to note when utilizing upper-body plyometric exercises. When high forces are placed on the upper body, the elbows will tend to point more anteriorly than is optimal. This is mainly due to the body trying to compensate for the force applied to the upper body. It is important to teach the athlete to keep his or her elbows closer to the torso, allowing the shoulder to stay within their normal anatomical position. By properly understanding the common faults of upper-body plyometric exercises, the strength and conditioning professional will be more prepared to observe the mistakes and promptly make corrections during training sessions.

28. B: During metabolic conditioning training, it is important to understand the various piece of equipment. Most equipment will allow the strength and conditioning professional to increase or decrease the resistance of the machine to change the intensity of the work. The rowing machine is equipped with the ability to increase or decrease air flow into the machine. This ability allows the strength and conditioning professional the ability to adjust the intensity of the machine.

29. A: Understanding the reasoning behind a general warmup is important for the strength and conditioning professional. During a general warmup, core temperature increases, circulation to muscles increases, and range of motion about the major joints increases.

30. D: During every exercise, there is a portion of the movement where the force will peak. This portion of the movement is termed the sticking point, and the athlete should learn to exhale during this time. Having a basic understanding of when the sticking point is during each exercise will allow the strength and conditioning professional to accurately cue the athlete through each exercise. Often, faulty movement patterns will occur during the sticking point because this point involves the most force on the athlete's body, so fatigue and compensatory mechanisms are common.

31. D: During plyometric training, after the energy is loaded into the muscle and tendons, there will be a brief period when the body changes direction and the muscle action shifts from eccentric to concentric work. This period is termed the amortization portion of the exercise. Although this could be considered an isometric portion of the exercise, the common terminology in plyometric training is amortization. Once the brief amortization period occurs, the muscles will start concentrically contracting.

32. C: Slight flexion of the knee (around 5-10 degrees) will prevent terminal knee extension and keep the knees in a healthy joint angle range. Although terminal knee extension can sometimes be a safe position during strength training, it is not considered to be safe in a conditioning training session where repetitive fatigue will occur. It is important to adjust the seat according to the athlete's anthropometry.

33. D: The only way to ensure proper breathing mechanics are employed during high-intensity anaerobic conditioning activities is to increase the length or frequency of rest periods when the athlete begins to fatigue. When fatigue occurs, the shoulders will begin to round forward, placing the athlete in a position where the aerobic system will be compromised. Understanding appropriate work-to-rest ratios for the goals of the training session is important when programming anaerobic conditioning activities.

34. C: Although a general warmup is important to perform before any stretching activity, it is not a benefit of static stretching. The main benefits of static stretching include increasing the range of motion of the joints, enhancing recovery, and serving as part of a corrective or rehabilitation program when done properly.

35. C: Knees caving in during hip, knee, and ankle free-weight exercises is a common mistake observed in many training sessions. Having the ability to correct this common flaw is important in ensuring a safe and effective training environment. Although the chest should be high during the entire execution of the movement, this verbal cue would not have any benefit for the stated flaw. By cueing the athlete to maintain outward pressure and ensure proper knee tracking, the hips will stay engaged and the athlete will correct the mistake of having the knees cave in during the movement.

36. D: The segments that comprise lower-limb sprinting mechanics include the eccentric braking period, the concentric propulsive phase, the recovery phase, and the ground preparation phase. Although the acceleration phase is a segment of sprinting mechanics, it is not a phase of the lower-limb mechanics.

37. A: Proper arm action is important during walking, jogging, and running exercises. As the right leg is coming forward, the left arm should be coming forward, and as the left leg is coming forward, the right arm should be coming forward. Natural movement at the shoulder joint is needed when utilizing these types of exercises. Throughout arm action, the elbow should stay flexed around 90 degrees and the hands should be in a relaxed position. The hands should come as high as the chest or sternum during the upward motion and back down to the lateral hip in the downward motion. By maintaining the full range of motion at the shoulder joint, the efficiency of the movement will increase.

38. A: When starting, the athlete should either be in an upright position, in a downward position in a three- or four-point stance, or in a downward position set in starting blocks. When the athlete is in any of the downward positions, the lead leg should be flexed to around 90 degrees and the trailing leg should be flexed to around 130 degrees. When starting, the athlete should focus on applying maximum force through the ground with both feet to propel his or her body forward horizontally. Within the first couple of strides, the athlete will transfer the force from horizontal displacement to gradual vertical displacement.

Program Design

Based upon an athlete's health status, training age, fitness, skill level, and training goals, the strength and conditioning professional must design an appropriate training programs that will maximize performance and minimize injury risk.

The most effective resistance and conditioning training programs for athletes are those that account for the unique needs of the individual. The strength and conditioning professional must design an athlete's optimal program that maximizes the benefits and minimizes the risk of injuries by taking a thorough inventory of the athlete's health status, training age, fitness, skill level, and training goals and developing the program accordingly. In implementing a comprehensive program that includes cardiovascular, power, speed, strength, flexibility and agility training, a strength and conditioning professional can provide an athlete with a well-rounded program that targets that athlete's specific goals and physiological needs. Resistance training and conditioning are, arguably, the most essential elements of an exercise training program for all populations. Regardless of the age, health condition, physical limitations, or fitness goals of the athlete, the resistance training portion of a strength and conditioning program can provide an athlete with countless health benefits including greater bony density and resistance against fractures, improved cardiovascular function, retainment of muscle mass with aging, better mood, and a higher metabolic rate.

Benefits of exercise training not only help alleviate physical issues and prevent the development of health conditions, but also improve athletes' quality of life. There are several resistance training techniques and program formats that can be utilized to incorporate this essential training into a comprehensive weekly exercise program. Any athlete (regardless of restrictions, limitations, specializations, or capabilities) can reap the benefits that these multi-functional exercises provide. Specific exercises can afford strength and conditioning benefits, cross-training capabilities, sport-specific improvements, and overall health improvements for the entire body. The ultimate goal is to maximize the benefit to each of the major muscle groups by rotating the strength and conditioning routine accordingly, providing each muscle and muscle group with a challenging routine that maximizes its potential and ability to contribute to optimal performance. Through deliberate programming techniques, specific muscle groups can be addressed via varied resistance training exercises in a "staggered" format. This can make even the minimum two-day recommendation sufficient in inducing strength and function improvements of the musculoskeletal system.

Incorporating Various Training Methods and Modes

Different Types of Training Methods and Modes

Free Weight Training Equipment
Free weights, such as barbells, dumbbells, kettlebells, and weight plates, are frequently used for resistance training exercises. These pieces of equipment are convenient, transportable, and versatile in their applications in exercises targeting any major muscle group. With a wide weight range available in many increments of weight, free weights can accommodate any athlete's unique restrictions or requirements, and be utilized as a tool for stability, strengthening, or muscle-building. As an athlete progresses in his or her proficiency and mastery of exercises, many free weight exercises can be made more challenging with the simple addition of weight or the manipulation of maneuvers that add a new level of difficulty. Safe preparations that include proper instruction and a demonstration of technique will help ensure that the free-weight resistance training of a strength and conditioning program will promote the athlete's healthy

achievement of program goals while reducing or eliminating the possibility of injury or harm. Consider the following sample free weight workout for beginners:

Basic Free Weights Workout for Beginners:
Do three sets of 8-12 reps for each exercise, or modify this number according to your fitness level.

Upper Body:

- Bench Press (chest and arms). Lay on a flat or incline bench press. Grip the barbell with the hands shoulder-width apart. Bring the barbell down to your chest, then push back up to full arm extension.

- Military Press (shoulders and arms). Done either sitting or standing. Hold either a barbell or two dumbbells at shoulder-height. Press the weight up and overhead to full arm extension, then lower the weight back down to the starting position.

- Barbell Row (arms and back). Stand with your feet slightly wider than shoulder-width apart and grip the barbell, which should be on the floor, with your hands close to the outside of each leg. Bend your knees slightly and hinge the torso forward from the hips to initiate the starting position. Do not round your back. From there, pull the barbell up to your chest, then control the decent back down to a hang.

Core:

- Deadlift (hamstrings and glutes). Begin with your feet hip-width apart, standing in front of a barbell that is resting on the ground. Bend your knees and hinge forward at the hips to grip the barbell, then straighten your knees and stand upright, bringing the barbell off the ground. It is important to keep your back straight and the barbell close to your legs while deadlifting. The bar should almost skim the shins in its path.

- Decline Sit-Up (core). Lay with your back against a decline bench, holding a small dumbbell in each hand. Place your hands where you feel comfortable for sit-ups (across the chest, behind the head, etc.), and perform your sit-ups as you normally would.

Lower Body:

- Back Squat (glutes, legs, core). At the squat rack, place the barbell over your shoulders, squeezing your shoulder blades together to make a shelf for the weight with your upper back. Holding that in place, bend your knees and squat to parallel or below parallel, then rise back up.

- Power Clean (legs, core). Begin the lift with a deadlift movement, bringing the barbell from the ground up to a standing position. Then, with the help of a hip-thrust, bring the weight up to your shoulders, rotating your hands and arms underneath the bar, and catching it with a slight dip in the knees.

- Lunges (glutes, hamstrings, quads). Stand and hold a dumbbell in each hand with your arms at your sides. Step forward with one foot, bending your front knee to a 90-degree angle, lowering yourself down until your back knee lightly brushes the floor before standing up.

Resistance Machines

Resistance machines provide strength and conditioning professionals and athletes with valuable way to conduct resistance training with specific structural support. Whether an athlete requires adaptive training or wants to isolate specific muscles or muscle groups, resistance machines can offer a unique approach to resistance training exercise that can only be provided by strategically-designed machinery and devices. Pulley systems, cams, hydraulics, friction-based machines, air-assisted technology, and even tubing-based machines can all be utilized in a versatile resistance training exercise program that can improve the strength, endurance, size, and power of an athlete's major muscle groups. Benefits of the basic resistance training program can be accelerated with the use of resistance training machines in populations who present health conditions or physical limitations by providing support and assistance in the posture, execution, and performance of an exercise. With illustrations demonstrating the proper use on each machine and the muscles it targets, resistance machines provide an added benefit to an athlete: After being instructed by a strength and conditioning professional about proper technique and execution, as is required initially, the athlete can feel confident in utilizing machines without assistance following the initial demonstration. Moreover, a spotter is not necessary with certain lifts that are mandatory when using free weights, so athletes can train independently when their schedule or budget doesn't allow for personalized or partner-based training as frequently as they need to strength train. Resistance machine exercises can also be included in a program as an athlete progresses, with the addition of weight, changes in posture, or manipulation of mechanics to increase the difficulty or resistance.

Plyometrics

Plyometrics approaches to resistance training exercise programming can provide an athlete with valuable health and fitness benefits without the need for equipment, facility space, or machines. Relying only on strategic exercises that utilize the body's own weight and positioning for resistance, the strength and conditioning professional and athlete can achieve the same benefits afforded by more traditional "weight training," but in any environment and at any time that the athlete finds suitable. While this approach to resistance training may be appealing to many coaches designing an athlete's program, the factors that should be considered are the athlete's age, experience, physical restrictions, capabilities, injury risk factors, and training goals, as each of these factors will allow or prohibit certain exercises. Strength and conditioning professionals who are designing a program for experienced, healthy athletes can determine the baseline of an athlete's expertise and ability, implement several plyometric exercises, and manipulate certain factors such as body placement, mechanics of movements, hold times, etc., in order to create a program that continues to challenge the muscles and muscle groups over time.

Speed/Sprint Training

Speed/sprint training come center stage in resistance and conditioning program design when an athlete is motivated to improve their performance and speed to benefit overall health, specific health goals, or sport-specific goals. While considering the athlete's age, previous experience in the movements and mechanics of sprinting, capabilities and restrictions, and training goals, multiple speed and sprint training exercises can be incorporated into a successful individualized training program. With restrictions taken into consideration, a strength and conditioning professional can present an athlete with accommodations and suggestions that can encourage effective speed training without inducing a significant risk of injury. By ensuring the athlete understands the mechanics of the movement and observing his or her performance so that it can be ceased if faulty mechanics occur at any point, a strength and conditioning professional can safeguard an athlete's health and maximize benefits of any and all exercises performed.

Interval Training

Interval training is simply a program design that includes intervals of high-intensity and low-intensity workouts that are used in succession to maximize an athlete's cardiovascular, muscular, and overall exercise performance endurance. With consideration of an athlete's age, abilities, restrictions, and health status, an appropriate training program can be designed that implements safe intervals of high- and low-intensity exercises that maximize benefit and minimize risk. Regardless of age, an athlete's major considerations in terms of interval training should be his or her health status and limitations. With high-intensity workouts falling into an anaerobic domain, athletes who have heart conditions, respiratory dysfunction, and a tendency to "push through" pain should all be considered high-risk for high-intensity varieties of interval training.

Agility Exercises

Agility exercises are essential in a training program for most sports, and every strength and conditioning professional should be determined to include these exercises where appropriate. Regardless of age, sex, skill level, or experience, any athlete should be presented with exercises that can maximize their agility (even on the smallest scale) in order to maximize their exercise benefits, while also promoting the very skills necessary to function successfully in daily life activities. While younger populations, as well as those who may have restrictions, should begin a program that incorporates beginner exercises that focus on balance, quick movements, and hand-eye coordination, athletes who are experienced can be introduced to resistance training exercises that incorporate bursts of movement that require agility and strength. As with all resistance training program designs, agility exercises should only be incorporated into a program after considering the athlete's age, health status, and abilities.

Aerobic Exercise

Aerobic exercise programs can provide an athlete with a multitude of training benefits that not only assist in the mastering of sports-specific goals or overall training-performance goals, but can also improve the athlete's overall health by bettering cardiovascular functioning, respiratory capacity, bone health, and muscular endurance. With the plentiful benefits of these exercises that include walking, jogging, running, swimming, biking, etc., an athlete's restrictions in terms of age, health status, and capabilities play a very small role in factoring aerobic activity inclusion in one's program. While high-impact exercises such as running may be suitable for those with minimal restrictions, an aerobic exercise of the low-impact variety (such as swimming) can yield just as many benefits for someone who has sustained an injury or has similar restrictions. By assessing an athlete's abilities, restrictions, and preferences, a strength and conditioning professional can successfully incorporate aerobic exercise into an athlete's training program in a healthy way.

Flexibility Exercises

Flexibility exercises are often considered as a warmup or cool-down activity that is only incorporated into a routine to prepare for a workout or to reduce soreness following an exercise routine. While both of these applications are necessary and helpful to all athletes, incorporating flexibility exercises into a program helps an athlete elongate and strengthen the elastic and inelastic fibers of muscles and connective tissues, engage muscle groups that may be neglected due to restrictions, and maximize range of motion (ROM) for improved sport performance and ease of daily life activities. An athlete's age, health status, and physical limitations can all assist a strength and conditioning professional in identifying the areas in which flexibility training can be most beneficial. The strength and conditioning professional should consistently observe the athlete's performance and inquire about tightness and soreness for indications of flexibility improvements.

Combinations of Various Training Methods and Modes to Reach a Certain Goal or Outcome

By incorporating a number of training methods and modes into an athlete's resistance and conditioning training program, a strength and conditioning professional can provide a progressive routine that includes variety and new, challenging, and exciting components that can help achieve specific goals while improving his or her overall health. With an appropriate rotation of exercises that focus on improving muscular endurance, hypertrophy, strength, power, and aerobic endurance, an athlete can gradually progress through a systematically-designed training program that fully encompasses the varied exercise components that yield optimal health and performance. This program should include regular assessments designed to gauge the athlete's improvement and reevaluate the suitability of the exercises (and their associated movements, weight, sets, and repetitions) in supporting the athlete's consistent progression toward his or her goals. While many of these modes of exercise may seem to be categorized so as to achieve certain goals, or focus on certain aspects of goals, these modes and methods can be interchangeably incorporated in a training program to keep varying the stimulus on the body, which encourages constant adaptation and minimizes plateaus.

To vary the modes of a workout, the strength and conditioning professional and athlete can utilize some basic applications that help ensure that the precise modes of each exercise routine promote balance and progression throughout the training program. Each session should keep the following in mind, regardless of the actual goals and exercises in the session:

Lever Length

By conveying the importance of lever length to athletes, the strength and conditioning professional can manipulate the most basic exercises in order to maximize their intensity and overall benefit. Understanding some basic biomechanical principles can assist in making any exercise harder or easier. If the goal is to make an exercise more challenging, the weight can be moved farther away from the fulcrum. Alternately, if the goal is to make the exercise less challenging, the weight should be moved closer to the fulcrum.

For example, the basic plank is an effective exercise that can be implemented into novice, intermediate, and expert training programs. Lifting one arm and placing it either in front of or stretched out beside the body increases the intensity of the exercise.

Balance

The better an athlete's ability to balance, the more safely and efficiently he or she will master mechanics and progress through fitness challenges and daily life activities with ease. Incorporating various modes of exercise that challenge athletes' balance skills, and improve their kinesthetic awareness will not only increase the challenge of a particular exercise, but also improve athletes' speed of mastering future workouts. Maintaining or improving balance is particularly important with elderly athletes as risk of fracture increases with age, due to reductions in bone mineral density. Balance should be incorporated into a training program, but should not detract from the athlete's primary goal.

Maintaining Focus

Throughout an exercise, an athlete should be constantly reminded to maintain focus. With a determination to be focused on the mechanics of an exercise, each part of an action can be performed with maximal effort for maximal benefit. Each action should be performed with precision; encourage athletes to maintain focus on their mechanics, breathing, and the anticipated physical outcomes of the exercises that are incorporated into their exercise training programs.

Repetition Manipulation

One common technique that can be used in exercise training programs is repetition manipulation. The number of sets and repetitions of certain exercises can be easily manipulated to optimize an athlete's training. For example, the squat can be used for any goal with a manipulation of repetitions:

- Complete sets of 1-5 repetitions for developing power
- Complete sets of 6-10 repetitions for muscle development
- Complete sets of 10+ repetitions optimize building muscle endurance

Time Under Tension (TUT)

The nomenclature for each phase of the lift is "eccentric—pause—concentric—pause" (all in seconds). A lift with a 4 x 1 x 0 tempo would equate to a 4-second eccentric motion, a 1-second pause, an explosive concentric, and no pause at the completion. The general rule is that the longer the time under tension, the more muscle damage produced, which maximizes muscle development. For example, strength exercises utilizing the TUT method require an explosive concentric contraction and a controlled or nonexistent eccentric (the weight is dropped as per a competition deadlift).

Weight

There are a number of variables to be considered when determining the weight used for exercises in a training program. Whether an athlete has specific health or fitness goals, struggles with inadequate fitness abilities or mechanical control, or has difficulty mastering certain exercises, the weight included in his or her unique exercise prescription will consistently require monitoring and changing throughout the progression of the program. To emphasize benefits, the goal should always be to challenge the athlete throughout the workout.

Additional Modes of Exercise

With multiple tools that can be utilized in exercise programs, there are a near infinite number of exercise modifications that are available to help an athlete attain a goal. With an athlete's abilities and capabilities kept in mind, the addition of BOSU balls, ropes, tires, kettlebells, etc., can be used to provide a consistent challenge to muscle groups and keep things everchanging.

Take, for example, the kettlebell. Because the weight distribution isn't uniform (the weight is concentrated at the bottom) the bell generates more inertia farther away from the body. This forces the athlete to engage more muscle groups with greater force and resistance to control the mechanics of the exercise.

Stance

Although most training manuals will provide the age-old approach to "proper" stance as being straight back, soft knees, and feet placed shoulder-width apart, stance can—and should—be varied to manipulate the areas of the body receiving the pressure and workload throughout a movement.

- Split Stance: This is a good stance because it is generally easier on the back and allows the athlete to maintain a strong posture. The wider the split, the more balanced the athlete will be. Just make sure to change up the leading leg so the athlete gets the oblique muscle benefit on both sides.

- Kneeling: Doing double-duty, kneeling can provide a multifaceted effect by incorporating and engaging multiple muscle groups. If the athlete is able to perform shoulder presses or biceps curls, one example of multi-engagement is to instruct the athlete to kneel during the performance of the exercise and activate the core muscles as well. Spotting by the strength and conditioning professional should be constant throughout the exercise.

- Half-Kneeling: With a stance just between standing and kneeling, a great benefit can be provided to the glutes, hamstrings, and core.

- Wide Stance: A wide stance makes it easy for the athlete to balance. It also gives the adductors a nice stretch.

- Feet Close Together: The closer the feet are, the more challenging the exercise is for the core.

Eccentrics (Negatives)

A *negative* is a very slowly-controlled contraction that can cause a lot of muscle demand in a minimal number of sets and repetitions. Reserved for advanced athletes, the recommendation is to keep sets between 20 and 50% greater than 1RM since more weight can be tolerated on the eccentric portion of a lift than the concentric portion. Therefore, the weight can be greater than that used for 1RM. An eccentric usually lasts around 10 seconds and requires the strength and conditioning professional to be a spotter and assist in the athlete's concentric portion of the lift, since the weight used exceeds what the athlete can handle for that portion of the lift. Muscle soreness in the days after the workout is common.

Rest Periods

Rest periods allow oxygen, enzymes, and essential nutrients to circulate to and from the muscle groups being activated throughout the performance of an activity. While the rest periods can vary depending upon an athlete's level of fitness, fitness goals, and capabilities, the rest period variable is one that can be extremely advantageous when maximizing the gains of an athlete's training program. Most strength and conditioning professionals learn about rest periods and when to use each one when they write their exam, and then largely forget about them in practice.

- 0–45 seconds of rest is recommended when trying to increase endurance
- 45–90 seconds of rest is recommended in workouts designed to build muscle
- 90 seconds or more of rest is recommended for strength training
- 2–5 minutes of rest is recommended for power training

Loading

Every exercise in a training session is directly affected by those that preceded it. Loading schemes can increase or decrease the intensity of a workout, or be designed to focus on a particular muscle group. Two examples are pre-fatigue and post-fatigue. Pre-fatigue occurs when an exercise that exhausts a single muscle group is performed and is then immediately followed by a multi-joint exercise using that same group, which can be dangerous if the lifter isn't experienced. For example, it is not recommended for an athlete to perform hamstring curls before a deadlift unless the lifter has a couple years of lifting experience and no contraindications to hamstring work. Post-fatigue is when a multi-joint exercise is followed immediately by a single-joint movement that uses one of the main muscles of the initial multi-joint movement. For example, a deadlift followed by a hamstring curl would be considered post-fatigue. This loading scheme is often used when increasing intensity and volume in training programming.

Pauses

Momentum is a powerful way to generate force, and it should be incorporated when beneficial, but avoided in training programs or exercises when it may not be beneficial. A full pause before a concentric contraction can train an athlete to recruit larger motor units faster, which can be advantageous if the athlete is seeking power generation. This strategy can also be effective in helping elderly athletes recover from trips or avoid future falls. Pausing at different stages of the contraction can also increase the intensity by increasing TUT and forcing the muscle to work at weaker ranges for longer periods of time.

Muscular Endurance

When an athlete is enduring a training program, whether with the goal to improve performance in a specific sport or to improve in overall health and wellness, exercises that increase muscular endurance are extremely important. Defined as the ability of muscles and muscle groups to sustain repeated contractions against resistance for an extended period of time, muscular endurance applies to athletes in engaging in most sports as well as those with general fitness pursuits. Whether the specific exercises include squats, lunges, and leg presses; abdominal crunches or Russian twists; or pull-ups with added resistance and weight or push-ups, the exercises that can be implemented into any athlete's routine for increasing muscular endurance can be effective for all goals and objectives, while also improving the athlete's performance in other elements of the training program and contributing to his or her overall health.

Hypertrophy

While the general rule for workouts intended to increase an athlete's size (muscle hypertrophy) is to focus on lifting high weight for few repetitions, the athlete's baseline performance of preliminary exercises can be used to determine the proper selection of exercises and the appropriate number of repetitions and sets for each. With the major muscle groups targeted, a successful training program should include a routine that rotates the major muscle groups in such a way that each is worked at least once every 48–72 hours to prevent full recovery of the muscle fibers between workouts. The strength and conditioning professional should keep in mind that the recommendation for exercises geared toward hypertrophy should be included at least twice weekly, rest periods should last less than sixty seconds, and that the negative motion of an exercise should always be slower than the positive.

Strength

To perform any exercise correctly, adequate strength is required. Regardless of an athlete's age, health status, and capabilities, a successful strength routine can be developed with careful consideration and modifications of specific exercises. While an athlete suffering from obesity, injury, or a chronic condition may require less intense, low-impact strength-training exercises, many exercises can be implemented for the strengthening of specific muscles and major muscle groups. The consistent reevaluation of the performance and progression of an athlete's mastering of certain strength exercises will allow for new exercises or changes in weight and repetitions to keep the muscles and muscle groups constantly challenged. While more advanced athletes may start a program with a stronger baseline, the exercises incorporated in any training regimen can provide adequate resistance for muscle growth, lengthening, and strengthening. With strength training, the resistance load is generally high, while repetitions remain low; as an athlete progresses, weight can be increased gradually, and repetitions can fluctuate depending upon mastery of the exercise performance.

Power

Power training should be included for a variety of athletes, except those who have certain chronic conditions or injuries. Athletes with cardiac issues, respiratory dysfunction, those struggling with a present or pre-existing injury, and those who are pregnant may not be suited to traditional power exercises and should be instructed to engage in light-intensity power exercises (if at all) chosen specifically to cater to their unique condition. Power is also likely less of a focus for truly endurance-based athletes like marathoners, long-distance triathletes, and endurance swimmers than those who participate in anaerobic sports. For advanced athletes who have engaged in power exercises previously, a strength and conditioning professional can implement a number of elements, such as strength- and speed-related exercises including jumps, sprint starts, etc., that challenge the ability of a muscle to contract in explosive spurts repeatedly. With the anaerobic pathway being utilized in a number of these power training modes, athletes who are ill-equipped to engage in power-focused training programs should be observed carefully as low-level power exercises are introduced.

Aerobic Endurance

Aerobic endurance refers to the capability of the aerobic pathway to be activated and engaged throughout a long-duration exercise performance. When walking, jogging, swimming, and biking, an athlete's increase in respiration and heart rate is to be expected, and with increased aerobic endurance, the activities in which these physiological changes take place will require less effort and become easier to endure. By implementing cardiovascular activities that encourage increases in aerobic endurance, any athlete can benefit from a multitude of cardiovascular, respiratory, muscular, skeletal, and even cognitive benefits. By assessing an athlete's baseline capabilities, an appropriate training program can be designed that includes a minimum of two to three 20–30-minute cardiovascular activities per week to improve aerobic endurance. For more advanced athletes, a strength and conditioning professional can implement up to six days of cardiovascular training exercises performed for durations of 30–60 minutes or more.

Selecting Exercises

In the process of developing a training program for a particular athlete, the strength and conditioning professional should fully understand the athlete's age, objectives, abilities, experience, and ultimate training goals. A strength and conditioning professional can design an optimal exercise program that includes multifaceted exercises that encompass specific movement patterns. Considering the athlete's particular sport or predominant activity, specific muscle groups can be targeted via a variety of kinetic-chain-based exercises, injury-prevention exercises, and exercises that can help promote recovery. As with all other training program exercises, a strength and conditioning professional must ensure that each exercise is explained in full detail and demonstrated to the athlete, enabling the athlete to comprehend the goal of the exercise, the muscles engaged and targeted, the mechanics involved during each movement, and how to reduce the risk of injury.

Exercises Specific to Movement Patterns of a Particular Sport

Exercises should focus on strengthening and conditioning the areas relevant to the activities most commonly performed in that athlete's particular sport. The body and limb movement patterns, muscular involvement, the associated joints' range of motion should all be taken into consideration when selecting the appropriate sport-specific exercises for an athlete. Another key factor to keep in mind is that, especially in sports that require disproportionate training, exercises should promote strengthening and conditioning of the opposing muscles for optimal muscle balance. Exercises that can emulate the precise activity or sport technique and can be assimilated into the athlete's performance when engaging in the actual sport or activity should be incorporated. Commonly referred to as the SAID principle, this transference of training to performance is a specificity concept: Specific Adaptation to Imposed Demands. By identifying the imposed demands and incorporating appropriate exercises that mimic those demands, a strength and conditioning professional can support an athlete's performance in training while engaging in the sport of focus.

Exercises Based Upon the Number or Type of the Involved Muscle Groups

When designing a training program that includes a multitude of exercises with unique training outcomes, a strength and conditioning professional should acknowledge that some varieties of exercises will be more beneficial based on an athlete's capabilities and needs. Using four basic categories of exercises (power, core, assistance, and structural), a strength and conditioning professional can maximize benefit and minimize injury while improving an athlete's sport-specific abilities and techniques. While structural movements are the most common in that they require stabilization of the spine bearing the load, full-body engagement should be considered. Incorporation of all major muscle groups and engagement of supporting muscles will maximize the benefit of the power exercises by adding an explosive component. Equating to a high-impact exercise that is often performed by seasoned athletes, these training programs can incorporate everything necessary to benefit and improve an athlete's success. Strength and conditioning professionals should ensure that exercises that engage the different major muscle groups are rotated in such a way that they allow adequate time for rest (the of which varies depending upon fitness goals–aerobic excellence versus hypertrophy), and that assistance muscles that further support the proper performance and execution of exercises prescribed are addressed as well.

Structural
Directly or indirectly loads the spine, but also recruits muscles for stabilization and proper posture during performance (example: deadlift)

Power
When appropriate for an athlete's sport-specific training, power exercises are those that involve the performance of a structural exercise performed very quickly or explosively (example: snatch)

Core
Recruits one or more of the body's major muscle groups (shoulders, chest, back, thighs, or hips)

Assistance
Recruits smaller muscle areas (abdominal muscles, upper arms, forearm, lower back, and lower legs)

Exercises Based Upon the Type of Kinetic Chain Movement

Kinetic chain movements are those in which the body's joints and segments all work together by having an effect on one another synergistically. When one joint and its associated segment/limb is moved, it effects another joint and segment, causing a chain of events. This chain of events is known as the *kinetic chain*. There are two kinds of kinetic chain movements: open and closed. In *open kinetic chain exercises*, the segment (a foot or hand) furthest from the body is not fixed to an object or the ground (for example, on a leg curl machine), while *closed kinetic chain exercises* require the segment to be fixed or stationary (for example, a squat). By implementing a combination of these two kinetic chain formats, a strength and conditioning professional can manipulate and isolate specific muscle groups and joints, and do so with or without assistance; machines that can provide hydraulic assistance can alleviate the impact and pressure of weight when certain athletes require such accommodations. Otherwise, a closed kinetic chain can place emphasis on the core, upper and lower extremities, etc. The correct choice often depends upon the goals of the athlete and the strength and conditioning professional's determination of which kinetic chain movements are most beneficial.

Exercises to Minimize Injury Potential

While preparing an athlete's training program, a strength and conditioning professional should always incorporate exercises that minimize injury potential. With information about an athlete's specific sports and activities, a strength and conditioning professional can identify the most commonly stressed and/or injured muscles, tendons, and joints, helping to determine the areas of the body that should receive additional attention in terms of exercises designed to minimize injury. By including exercises that require muscle balance, all muscles receive adequate training and attention, which can minimize atrophy and performance weaknesses. In these exercises, the *agonistic muscles* are those causing the movement, while the *antagonistic muscles* are those opposing or supporting the agonistic (for example, hamstrings versus quadriceps, upper versus lower).

Exercises to Promote Recovery

Throughout the development of a training program, a strength and conditioning professional should include exercises that promote recovery. Many exercises, whether aerobic or anaerobic, can result in lactic acid buildup in the muscles that can lead to muscle soreness and stiffness. This post-workout discomfort can be avoided if appropriate exercises and routines that are specifically intended to promote recovery are implemented. By stretching, flexing, massaging, and lengthening the muscles involved (both the major muscle groups and supporting muscles), the lactic acid buildup can be gradually released and dispelled via the body's metabolic systems. With foam rollers, yoga poses, stretches, and a multitude of flexibility exercises, recovery exercises can be chosen that fit the athlete's needs and preferences.

In addition to exercises that can promote recovery, extensive scientific studies have observed the lifestyle habits that contribute to faster recoveries between exercise sessions and have deemed a number of habits helpful. Regardless of age, fitness level, or fitness goal, the importance of adequate recovery for optimal gains cannot be stressed enough. If an athlete needs additional motivation or ideas of ways to rest and recover, the strength and conditioning professional can share these options:

1. Regulate Sleep Routines. It has long been determined that sleep has a major impact on health. Regarding the quality and quantity of sleep, one of the most important things to ensure an athlete's optimal performance is to recommend maximizing sleep for overall health. Hormonal balance, better focus, increased fat-loss, and improved endurance all result from improved sleep patterns.

2. Listen to Music. While pushing through a challenging cardio routine can be alleviated with high-tempo music, researchers have determined that listening to low-tempo music following high-endurance workouts improves recovery in speed and intensity. This means an athlete can reap benefits faster and return to activity more quickly and ably.

3. PM Protein. During the eight-hour break that sleep provides the body, the muscles, tissues, and cells are all in repair mode. By providing ample sources of protein, such as low-fat cottage cheese or turkey breast, the body can reap the massive benefits of protein-rich PM snacks throughout the evening while it works through sleep.

4. AM Carbs and Protein. After a good night's rest, the body needs nutrients to recharge. High-protein breakfasts with ample complex carbohydrates can give muscles the necessary ingredients to start rebuilding and may reduce food cravings later in the day. By providing the body with a combination of energy-producing carbohydrates and muscle-repairing protein, the body's cells, organs, and systems can all function optimally.

5. Cherry and Pomegranate Juices. With impressive amounts of vitamins, minerals, and potent antioxidants, cherry and pomegranate juices provide the body with micronutrients that not only maximize recovery, but restore cells, organs, and systems for future workouts.

6. Hydrate. Exercising while dehydrated can cause greater damage to muscles and reduce the body's ability to repair itself. Before reaching for sports drinks, however, know that water is often enough for many individuals looking to replenish fluids. Always remember that signs of thirst indicate the onset of dehydration. If there are signs of thirst, ensure that the daily recommendation of eight 8-oz. glasses of water is being consumed, with more during and after exercise.

7. Eliminate Alcohol. Not only is alcohol a depressant, it also poses hazardous risks to the brain and body. With empty calories that contribute to weight gain, heart complications, performance issues, and depression being byproducts of alcohol consumption, water and all-natural alternatives are far better than any alcoholic beverage.

8. Massage. Not only does a massage help relieve tension, it also helps release the buildup of acidic metabolic byproducts in muscle fibers throughout workouts and afterward. Massages can help release built-up enzymes and acids that accumulate throughout workouts and recovery, and help metabolize the biological byproducts.

9. Pre-Workout Protein. Amino acids are the building blocks of tissue, and protein gives bodies enough to rebuild and maintain muscles damaged during workouts. Having a little protein before working out can trigger an athlete's body to start *muscle synthesis* (repairing and building more muscle) throughout, and even after hitting the weights.

10. Post-Workout Protein. While a protein-rich snack can get the body ready for a workout, sipping on a protein smoothie or eating a protein-filled meal after a workout can ensure the body has enough fuel to keep on rebuilding throughout the day.

11. Nap. Researchers have determined that a short nap lasting between 20 and 30 minutes taken midday can provide the body and brain with restorative rest that helps replenish hormones and recharge the body's cells and systems.

12. Appropriate Muscle Rest. While many strength and conditioning professionals recommend a certain number of days between workout for rest and reparation, there is no one-size-fits-all recommendation. To improve stamina, maximize benefits, and minimize the risk of injury, strength and conditioning professionals and athletes should be in constant communication about rest period needs.

Applying the Principles of Exercise Order

There are seven generally accepted principles of exercise order that are crucial in a training program designed to support an athlete in progressing toward and achieving a fitness goal. These principles of exercise order include individuality, specificity, progression, overload, adaptation, recovery, and reversibility.

Individuality refers to each individual athlete's unique response to training, in that some athletes are able to endure and adapt when presented with advanced training exercises quicker than others. Individual differences can be due to a number of factors including genetic predisposition, muscle fiber types, age, abilities, lifestyle factors, and health status.

Specificity refers to an athlete's need for exercises that help accelerate skills and abilities specific to his or her sport or activity. Training should be focused on major muscle groups commonly utilized in the performance of the sport or activity. Exercises chosen to be included in an athlete's training program should focus on those major muscle groups, and on the supporting muscle groups as well. Engaging in exercises that mimic the movements of the athlete's sport or activity also helps improve ability and performance.

Progression refers to an athlete's training program's methodical building or "challenge" to consistently maintain a requirement of effort that improves strength, endurance, stamina, and ability. Using an analogy of building blocks, a strength and conditioning professional can convey the principle of progression. By explaining that each successful achievement in mastering a skill, speed, or time allows for a progressive goal to be set that can replace the already-achieved goal. With each progression, the athlete acquires better abilities that can be improved upon again and again as the progression leads to successful achievement of his or her ultimate training goal.

Overload is the principle of consistently adding resistance to an athlete's training exercises and routines in an effort to improve muscle adaptation and avoid plateaus. With the maintenance of the same resistance, muscle fibers become accustomed to the routine and fail to progress. The ideal goal is to consistently successfully progress through a program to the next level of performance. With an overload of too much weight or effort, the risk of injury increases, so constant awareness and progressive overload should be the focus of this aspect of exercise selection.

Adaptation is the principle of the body's natural ability to grow accustomed to certain routines. Whether it be a movement, method, mode, weight, or performance of an exercise, the body will automatically adapt to increase in efficiency, but require less effort. In order to avoid adaptation in this sense, the strength and conditioning professional and athlete should work together in consistently restructuring the exercises and training program to vary the muscle mechanics of an exercise while gradually increasing intensity and duration. With slight changes, massive gains can be achieved.

Recovery refers to the time between exercises that allows the body to rest and repair itself. During a workout, the muscle fibers undergo microtears and require adequate nutrients, blood flow, and hormonal balance, all of which are only optimized with rest. Whether hours and days between major muscle group work or days and weeks between high-intensity training are needed, the strength and conditioning professional and athlete must maintain a disciplined program that includes periods of rest for adequate recovery. Reducing the risk of overworking and injury, recovery is a must in proper training program planning.

Reversibility is the principle that is most often referred to with the saying, "Use it, or lose it!" When training for a goal, the maximum effort that is put forth to achieve that goal becomes less necessary when the goal has been achieved, or when that goal is no longer pertinent in a training program. For instance, the training for athletes during the off-season is far less intense; thus, the effort required is also far less. While the effort may not remain the same, athletes should be encouraged to maintain a proper training program that ensures the muscles and systems do not atrophy. With a reduction in strength, conditioning, stamina, and ability, an athlete can jeopardize his or her future performance with the reversibility that takes place with the failure to maintain a proper program.

Order of Exercises Based on the Training Goal

In an effort to maximize the benefits of a training program, the strength and conditioning professional should plan an order of exercises that takes into consideration the goal of the particular athlete. For athletes, total body training in which all major muscle groups are targeted with one to two exercises per training session can yield maximum results in strength and conditioning. For powerbuilders and bodybuilders, an "upper-lower split" format that engages just the upper major muscle groups during one session and the lower body muscle groups in another session is ideal, allowing the muscle groups of each session's training to have short periods of rest between workouts. The muscle group split approach allows a strength and conditioning professional to design a training program for the average athlete by focusing on opposing muscle groups, such as biceps and glutes, in one session, followed by hamstrings and abdominals in another. By taking the athlete's training goal into consideration, the strength and conditioning professional can develop an order of exercises for every training session that maximizes the benefits and improves the athlete's progression through the training program.

Variations in Exercise Orders

By varying the order of exercises in training sessions, a strength and conditioning professional can ensure that the athlete's execution of the planned exercises is performed correctly, with adequate energy and stamina, and with limited risk of injury. Exercises performed in the initial phase of a training session are performed with less fatigue, allowing for ideal performance and maximum effort. Higher-intensity exercises should always be performed prior to the lower-intensity exercises, allowing for optimal performance for each. In general, large muscle groups should be targeted first, and the supporting smaller muscle groups can follow. Also, multiple-joint exercises should always be performed initially, followed by single-joint exercises such as leg extensions, allowing for support and less resistance as the athlete's energy declines.

Variations in Exercise Modes

When varying the exercise routines in an athlete's training program, the strength and conditioning professional should consider the benefits of a number of exercise modes. With explosive training, an athlete can maximize their potential in speed and power, utilizing anaerobic energy pathways that reduce the dependency on oxygen. With strength training exercise implementations, an athlete can gain strength, stamina, and endurance that targets specific muscle groups and improves the muscles' ability to perform. With the introduction of warmups and cooldowns prior to and after the workout, the athlete can benefit from increased energy and flexibility, which results from muscle fibers and tendons having the opportunity to "wake up" prior to engaging in a physical activity; conversely, the cooldown allows the muscles to stretch and release metabolic waste products that can lead to stiffness and soreness following physical activity. With energy system training prioritization, an aerobic platform provides a base from which athletes can build upon with sport-specific exercises that can easily transfer to their performance in their sport.

Determining and Assigning Exercise Intensities

Commonly referred to as the *FITT principle*, the four basic keys to designing the most beneficial training program for an athlete are Frequency, Intensity, Time, and Type. With each of these factors being considered in the design of a fitness training program, the strength and conditioning professional can effectively promote an athlete's successful progression throughout the program to accommodate the ultimate achievement of the athlete's health and fitness goals.

- *Frequency* refers to the number of days per week that each muscle group is trained. Depending upon the athlete's schedule, preference, and goals, the frequency can be manipulated to conform to his or her specific needs.

- *Intensity* (also referred to as *load*) refers to the amount of weight or resistance used for the exercise being performed. The *one-repetition maximum (1RM)* is the most commonly used assessment for determining the appropriate intensity.

- *Time* (also referred to as *volume*) refers to the repetitions and sets prescribed for each exercise (or the duration of aerobic efforts). A *repetition* is a single performance of an exercise's motion, such as the lifting and return to natural position of a weight. A *set* is the group of repetitions performed in succession without pause. Sets are interrupted with periods of rest, breaking sets into intervals. Ideally, the greater the load, the fewer the reps, while the lighter the load, the higher the number of reps.

- *Type* refers to the mode of the exercise. Whether the exercise falls into a category of muscular endurance, aerobic endurance, strength, power, or hypertrophy, countless exercises are available that will provide athletes with benefits that progress them toward their ultimate training goal.

Methods for Assigning an Exercise Load

One repetition maximum (1RM) is the greatest resistance or weight that can be moved through the full range of motion with proper posture and in a controlled manner for a single repetition. By either estimating an athlete's ability to perform a one repetition maximum or directly performing the test, the repetition max test can determine the *Repetition Maximum (RM)* to be used in consideration for future exercises. As an athlete increases his or her strength, power, and endurance, the increase in load and, thus, the change in the 1RM, will provide a progressive path toward successful goal accomplishment.

The Karvonen method for determining an athlete's ideal exercise heart rate is one of the easier applications to use in preparing and progressing through an effective training program. The *Karvonen formula*, devised by a Scandinavian physiologist, calculates the difference between the maximal heart rate and the resting heart rate, which is termed *heart rate reserve (HRR)*. From there, exercise intensities are determined by calculating certain percentages of the HRR added to the resting heart rate and using that heart rate as a target for the workout. For example, if an athlete is 20, he or she has an estimated maximal heart rate of 193 bpm ($207 - (0.7 \times age\ in\ years)$). If that athlete's resting heart rate is 55 bpm, the HRR is 138 bpm (193 – 55 bpm). Then, if the target maximal heart rate for a workout was 85% of the HRR, that athlete should strive to keep the heart rate at or below 172 bpm ((0.85×138 bpm) + 55 bpm).

Load or Exercise Heart Rate Based on the Training Goal

With the exercise training program in place, a strength and conditioning professional and athlete can work together to maximize benefits, minimize risk, and prepare to proceed through a program designed to help achieve successful goals that build upon one another until the ultimate fitness or health goal is realized. By monitoring an athlete's heart rate, the strength and conditioning professional and athlete can monitor progress, maintain focus on areas that need improvement, and accelerate training with suitable changes in mode, intensity, frequency, and duration of exercises.

With the widely accepted formula used to determine maximum heart rate as $220 - age\ in\ years$, or the alternative (and arguably, more accurate) $207 - (0.7 \times age\ in\ years)$, the percentage of the maximum heart rate should be determined for each individual athlete's unique health or fitness goal.

- Aerobic Endurance: 65–75% of maximum heart rate (MHR) for 12 or more reps
- Hypertrophy: 75–85% of maximum heart rate (MHR) for 6–12 reps
- Anaerobic: 85–90% of maximum heart rate (MHR) for 3–5 reps
- Strength: 85–90% of maximum heart rate (MHR) for approximately 6 reps
- Power: 90%+ of maximum heart rate (MHR) for 1–3 reps

Determining and Assigning Training Volumes

Outcomes Associated with the Manipulation of Training Volume

With each training program goal, the variation and progression of training volumes can support an athlete in successfully achieving maximum benefits from the exercise routine, as well as realizing his or her ultimate goals. While muscular strength exercises should include fewer than eight repetitions of heavier loads, higher repetitions of lighter loads are commonly prescribed for muscular endurance. Each of the training goals every unique athlete may have can be as varied as the athletes themselves, and so a strength and conditioning professional must assess the athlete's abilities and determine the most effective training volumes for the athlete's successful progression and ultimate achievement of his or her training program's goal.

Volume Based on the Training Goal

When training an athlete with a specific training goal—such as improving muscular endurance, aerobic performance, strength, power, or hypertrophy—there are several factors that must be taken into consideration when determining the volume for each exercise. When training for specific goals, the number of repetitions and sets, as well as the loads, must all be closely monitored throughout each session to ensure that the athlete is able to have each aspect of the exercise's volume changed appropriately as he or she progresses in fitness level.

Determining and Assigning Work/Rest Periods, Recovery and Unloading, and Training

Work/Rest Periods and Recovery

When preparing an athlete to engage in an effective fitness program, workloads, rest periods, recovery, and training frequency must all be determined. For the appropriate program that is designed specifically to assist in the accomplishment of a particular health, fitness, or athletic goal, it is imperative that the strength and conditioning professional conduct the correct assessments that aid in determining all of the critical elements involved. Taking into consideration that work periods vary depending upon the specific goal, the strength and conditioning professional should schedule sets, repetitions, weight loads, and rest periods very differently for an athlete whose goal is power than for an athlete whose goal is muscular endurance or strength training. The following are some pertinent guidelines to follow:

- *Muscular Endurance:* Include high repetitions with short rest periods of 0–90 seconds between sets; the weight required for work should increase gradually as the program progresses and the athlete reaches points of adaptation or "plateaus."

- *Hypertrophy:* Depending upon the athlete's fitness level and experience, the load, volume, and intensity may vary widely, but repetitions and sets are separated by shorter rest periods that range between 0 and 60 seconds.

- *Strength:* Strength training focuses on lower weight and higher repetitions with short rest periods of 0–90 seconds, depending on the athlete's level of fitness and mastery of the exercise. With strength training, the concern of adaptation should be considered at all times, ensuring that the athlete and strength and conditioning professional are in constant and consistent communication regarding assessing and determining if load, volume, or intensity should be adjusted.

Here is a sample workout for an athlete interested in increasing leg strength:

Exercise	Intensity* (8 RM)	Repetitions	Tempo	Sets	Volume
Barbell Front Squats	115 lbs.	8	2/1/1	4	3,680 lbs.
Barbell Deadlifts	155 lbs.	8	2/1/1	4	4,960 lbs.
Kettlebell Swings (Two-Hands)	50 lbs.	8	Explosive	4	1,600
Lateral Step-Ups	25 lbs.	8	1/1/1	4	800
Single-Leg Romanian Deadlift	25 lbs.	8	2/1/1	4	800
Total Session Volume					11,840 lbs.

*Intensity—the amount of weight used equals the athlete's 8-rep max for that lift.

- *Power:* In power training, the goal is to perform low repetitions with increasingly high weight, requiring 3–5 minutes between sets. As power-focused exercises are performed regularly throughout an exercise program, the athlete and strength and conditioning professional must anticipate the athlete's adaptation to weight loads and be prepared to restructure the program accordingly.

Training Frequency

With exercise training programming involving a number of factors, the strength and conditioning professional must take into account the athlete's level of fitness, goals, and appropriate exercise routine that will assist the athlete in achieving their ultimate fitness or health goal. With a wide variety of exercises that can be used to target the major muscle groups, the strength and conditioning professional can select the most challenging exercises for each. Those that help to improve the athlete's abilities and mastering of particular movements should be emphasized, but training frequency can also play a major role in the increasing the body's ability to achieve health and fitness goals faster.

Keeping in mind that the major muscle groups require the most time for repair after intense workouts, strength and conditioning professionals and athletes can coordinate the most beneficial training routine for muscular endurance, strength, power, metabolic conditioning, and recovery. By identifying the health or fitness goal of the athlete and assigning the appropriate frequency of workouts that are in most accordance with that specific goal, the athlete can reap massive benefits effectively and quickly with a program's success guaranteed.

Novice: New athletes who are unfamiliar with training routines, muscle mechanics of exercises, or mastering of specific exercise routines, should be trained with an "entire body" focus 2–3 days per week. Generally speaking, an athlete who has been training less than two or three months, with two or fewer sessions per week, is considered a novice. These athletes are in the beginning stages of training and have a low skill level.

Intermediate: Regardless of the goal for training, intermediate athlete (who are athletes who have been training at least three times per week for two months or more) are still between the novice and mastering stages of exercise performance, requiring constant and consistent evaluation and programming that allows for improvement in mastered exercises, while extra effort can be focused on areas in need of improvement. These athletes are able to perform three days of total-body workouts or four days of upper/lower body splits that train each major muscle group twice weekly.

Advanced: Advanced athletes have been training consistently for at least one year and completing around four sessions per week. This frequency can be increased to 4–6 days weekly, and they can focus on each major muscle group 1–2 times per week. The intensity of the workouts can also be increased. While these athletes still require constant, consistent supervision, evaluation, and assessment by the strength and conditioning professional, these advanced athletes may be able to endure an exercise program that includes two daily workouts that rotate major muscle groups throughout the week's progression. For example, pulling muscles may be the focus on Monday morning with a sprint workout on the track in the afternoon. Tuesday may have a long cardio bike ride in the morning followed by a session in the weight room in the afternoon focused on pushing muscles.

Determining and Assigning Exercise Progression

As athletes progress through their exercise training program, the strength and conditioning professional can progress the difficulty of the program in terms of mode, intensity, duration, and frequency. Each athlete's training routine should be created as per his or her specific health or fitness goals. The determination of an athlete's abilities and limitations as well as his or her mastery of the movement mechanics for each exercise should be taken into consideration when planning or reassessing an exercise program's components. Knowing that the body will adapt to exercises' intensities, durations, frequencies, etc., the strength and conditioning professional and athlete can work together to identify areas in which progression can be made. After all, progress is the ultimate goal of training. The athlete should remain focused on the fact that progress is made in different areas of the body at different rates and with different modalities of resistance. Over time, the athlete will be able to identify areas of strengths and weaknesses and be able to work with the strength and conditioning professional to determine a schedule and routine that maximizes benefit to all major muscle groups with the least effort, and without areas of need being adversely neglected.

Mode

Throughout the training progression, the strength and conditioning professional will assign an athlete exercises that require different mechanics to be performed by various major and supporting muscle groups. Once it is determined that specific muscle groups require more, or less, focus to perform at their optimal level, appropriate exercises will be assigned and replaced or improved upon according to the athlete's physiological and psychological responses.

The mode of exercise can alternate between free-weight, machine, and body-weight-related exercises as exemplified in the table below:

Muscle Area	Free-weight	Machine	Body-Weight
Chest	Supine Bench-Press	Seated Chest Press	Push-Ups
Back	Bent-Over Barbell Rows	Lateral Pull-Downs	Pull-Ups
Shoulders	Dumbbell Lat Raises	Shoulder Press	Arm Circles
Biceps	Barbell/Dumbbell Curls	Cable Curls	Reverse Grip Pull-Ups
Triceps	Dumbbell Kickbacks	Press-Downs	Dips
Abs	Weighted Crunches	Seated Abdominal Machine	Crunches/ Prone Planks
Quadriceps	Back Squat	Leg Extensions	Lunges
Hamstrings	Stiff-Leg Deadlifts	Leg Curls	Hip-Ups

Intensity

Whether training to run a marathon or attempting to increase one's one repetition maximum (1RM), an athlete's intensity of training is an imperative part of a successful program. With each athlete presenting unique goals and working from unique starting points or fitness levels, each athlete's exercise intensity should be evaluated and assigned on an individual basis. For the following goals, the novice-intermediate recommendation is provided as well as the advanced:

- Muscular strength: 60–70% of 1RM (novice-intermediate), 80–100% (advanced)
- Power: 30–60% 1RM for upper body, 0–60% for lower body
- Hypertrophy: 70–85% of 1RM (novice-intermediate), 70–100% of 1RM (advanced)
- Endurance: 70–85% of 1RM (novice-intermediate), 70–100% (advanced)

Duration

The fitness level and capabilities of each athlete should be considered throughout the exercise program planning. The baseline guidelines for novice, intermediate, and advanced athletes in terms of duration are provided below. From these baseline guidelines, the strength and conditioning professional and athlete should evaluate and reevaluate the athlete's progress to ensure that the appropriate exercises and durations are being included for optimal progress.

- Muscular strength: 1–3 sets of 8–12 reps (novice-intermediate), 2–6 sets of 1–8 reps (advanced)
- Power: 1–3 sets of 3–6 reps per exercise
- Hypertrophy: 1–3 sets of 8–12 reps (novice-intermediate), 3–6 sets of 10–12 reps (advanced)
- Endurance: 2–4 sets of 10–25 repetitions

Frequency

As with all of the elements of the exercise training program development, frequency must be taken into consideration. While the unique fitness goal of the athlete should dictate the direction and progression of the program, the strength and conditioning professional and athlete should consider the athlete's starting fitness level and progress from that point.

- Novice: Athletes should train the entire body 2–3 days per week

- Intermediate: Athletes should train three days for full-body workouts, or 4 days for upper/lower body split training

- Advanced: Athletes should train 4–6 days per week, training each major muscle group 1–2 times per week

- Elite Bodybuilders and Lifters: For these athletes, high frequency training is recommended, with two workouts per day, 4–5 days per week

Applying the Principles of Periodization

Periodization is the general approach to improving the fitness benefits and reducing the incidence of injury by systematically staggering "cycles" or periods of training.

Periodization

Hans Selye proposed the first model of periodization termed the *General Adaptation Syndrome*. Determining that biological stresses provided by training in athletes and fitness-oriented athletes produced benefits and consequences when orchestrated accordingly, he determined that overtraining over extended periods of time could lead to tissue damage, disease, and death. In order to avoid these detrimental outcomes, the concept of periodization was born and became an accepted approach to training athletes and non-athletes alike. By avoiding overtraining and systematically alternating routines to improve and benefit the performance of specific areas of technique and ability, high loads of training are alternated with decreased loads and higher intensities to improve speed, endurance, and strength throughout the cycles of periodization.

Many training variables can be manipulated in an attempt to optimize the exercise program: the number of sets per exercise, repetitions per set, the types of exercises, number of exercises per training session, rest periods between sets and exercises, resistance used for a set, type and tempo of muscle action (e.g., eccentric, concentric, isometric), and the number of training sessions per day and per week.

In a periodized exercise program, the terms *volume* and *intensity* are frequently used. In weight-training programs, *intensity* refers to the weight lifted relative to a maximal strength level (e.g., one-repetition maximum), or a multiple-repetition maximum (e.g., 10-repetition maximum). In a running or conditioning program, intensity is often used to describe a percentage of an age-predicted maximum heart rate or VO_2 max. In general, the higher the intensity, the lower the volume of a particular exercise or workout. *Training volume* refers to the total number of sets, reps, and exercises performed in a strength training program, and the distance and/or time of a conditioning program.

Training Variations Based on a Sport Season

Throughout training, methods including periodization can benefit an athlete by ensuring that the most appropriate training modes, intensities, durations, and volumes are used periodically to improve performance and minimize the risk of overtraining or injury. The periodization is divided into three cycles: the microcycle, mesocycle, and macrocycle.

- Microcycle: Seven days that include progressive overloading that prepares an athlete for more intense activities during the advanced stages of training.

- Mesocycle: Typically 3–4 weeks in length, the mesocycle is a specific time period in the training intended to reach a specific goal. While the mesocycle lasts 3–4 weeks, it is usually broken into a 21–28-day training period that consists of 21–23 training days and five days of rest.

- Macrocycle: This 52-week cycle gives strength and conditioning professionals and athletes a broad overview of the training program that will be broken into microcycles and mesocycles that comprise the entire macrocycle. While the macrocycle has the training program broken into high-intensity and low-intensity training periods that build up to the athlete's competition or peak season, strength and conditioning professionals and athlete should be in constant communication about the program's progression and inclusion of all four stages: endurance, intensity, competition, and recovery.

A Periodized Program Specific to the Athlete's Demands of a Sport, Position, and Training Level

While a periodized program needs to be outlined and designed with specifics that promote progress in the athlete's areas of need (i.e., stretching, rowing, throwing, kicking, etc.), the strength and conditioning professional and athlete should be sure to include total-body conditioning resistance training exercises that improve and maintain the athlete's conditioning and capabilities off-season, as well as during the competitive season. With specific focus on the athlete's sport requirements, the strength and conditioning professional and athlete can develop an optimal resistance and conditioning training program that not only prepares the athlete for the competition phase, but also maximizes the benefits to the athlete throughout the recovery and off-season phases as well.

The following table provides an example of the phases of a periodized program:

	Phases of the Periodized Program			
	Hypertrophy	Strength	Power	Peaking
Sets	2 – 4	2 – 5	3 – 5	1 – 3
Reps	8 – 20	4 – 8	3 – 5	1 – 3
Volume	High	High	Low	Low
Intensity	Low	Med High	High	Very High

The next table provides examples of combination routines that might be utilized in a strength training program:

Day 1	Day 2	Day 3
Squat or Leg Press	Lunges	Bench Press
Bench Press	DB Press	3 Position Pulls*
Pull-ups	DB Row	Squat
Step-ups	Leg Extension	Leg Curl
Incline DB Press	DB Press	Calf raises
Bent Over/Machine Row	Leg Curl	Superset Bicep Curls and Tricep Extensions
Romanian Deadlifts	Biceps	
Rotator-Cuff Circuit	Triceps	

The following table provides an example of upper-lower routines

Upper 1	Upper 2	Lower 1
Bench Press	Pull-Ups	Step-Ups
Incline Press	DB Bench Press	Lunges
Military Press (standing)	DB Rows	Squats
Triceps Extension	Incline DB Press	Leg Curls
Bent-Over Row	DB Shrugs	Romanian Deadlifts
Lat Pull-down	DB Triceps Extension	Plantar Flexion
Shrugs	DB Curls	Dorsi-flexion
Biceps Curls		

The following table provides an example of split routines:

Push	Pull	Push/Pull Combo
Bench Press	Cable/Pulley Row	Lunges
Squat	Deadlift	Incline DB Press
Military Press	Chin-Ups	Step Ups
Step Ups	Leg Curls	Upright Rows
Triceps Extension	High Pulls	Russian Deadlifts
Calf Raises	Biceps Curls	Biceps
Back Extensions	Crunches	Triceps
		Crunches with Twist

Designing Programs for an Injured Athlete During the Reconditioning Period

When designing a training program for an injured athlete during their reconditioning period, the strength and conditioning professional and athlete should ensure that the progression of the reconditioning process is understood and agreed upon. Taking time, effort, and patience to heal, the injured athlete can become frustrated with slow progress, restrictions in abilities, and pain. While recognizing all of these factors, both physical and psychological, that can interfere with an athlete's progress to optimal performance, there are a number of tools that can be utilized to help the communication between strength and conditioning professional and athlete to expedite recovery, minimize the risk of exacerbating the injury, and improve overall conditioning without causing more harm or dealing healing.

Types of Injuries

The following are categories of common injuries:

Macrotrauma: Broken bones are the most frequently thought of physical ramification of a macrotrauma, but this category of injuries also includes injured tendons, sprains, joint dislocations, and injuries from overuse. Macrotraumas are normally seen in acute injuries resulting from frequent overuse of muscles, joints, ligaments, tendons, and bones.

Dislocation: Complete or partial joint dislocations. The injuries cause the ends of bone to differ from their original positioning and can cause immediate or permanent damage, depending upon the speed and intensity of the healing process. The main concern with a dislocation is that the healing prescription must provide the surrounding tissues and ligaments with adequate support to return the injured areas to functional processes with limited intervention.

Contusion: Bruises can occur anywhere throughout the body, but most people associate these injuries with the aesthetic blue, black, purple, or green appearances that show on the skin following an injury. Specifically, a contusion is a specific afflicted area of tissue that has been damaged extensively, resulting in ruptures to capillaries, which allows blood to pool under the skin and form a bruise.

Strain: While these injuries seem minimal, ruptures and tears to the organs, ligaments, and tendons can have serious ramifications that not only limit or inhibit abilities and functions of organs, systems, and movement, but daily life activities as well.

Microtrauma: Overuse injuries are commonly seen in novice or expert athletes who push the limits. By adhering to an aggressive exercise training regimen that incorporates exercises and increases training volumes and loads gradually as an athlete's capabilities increase and improve, microtraumas can be avoided, or at least minimized.

Tendinitis: Inflammation of a tendon is a common injury when training for sports and conditioning purposes. While the strength and conditioning professional and athlete can stay clear on the current fitness level, point of success, and desired path to achieve success, there are a number of factors that can interfere. Overuse, infections, and chronic diseases are examples of causes of tendonitis. This injury can inhibit the full potential of an exercise training program and cause irreversible damage to the tendons and surrounding tissues.

Tissue Healing

After a musculoskeletal injury, there are generally three phases of tissue healing. Although severity of the injury within each phase may differ for each tissue type, all tissues follow the same basic pattern of healing.

First, the *inflammation phase* is characterized by pain, swelling, and redness, which occurs immediately after the injury and can last from several hours to a week or so. Collagen synthesis decreases and inflammatory cells migrate to the site of injury. The immediate area around the injury becomes hypoxic as the tissues, especially capillaries, are damaged. This environment causes further tissue death and signals the release of chemical mediators like bradykinin and histamine, which cause further edema. This swelling inhibits the function of contractile tissue, stimulates phagocytosis to rid the area of the damaged and dead tissue, and causes pain, due to sensory neuron activation.

Next, the *repair phase* occurs as the number of inflammatory cells decreases and healing starts to begin; it may last several weeks. Collagen fibers are produced but as they assemble at the site of the injury, they do so in a disorganized manner. This haphazard arrangement makes the connective tissue less strong because tissue strength is optimized when the collagen fibers are aligned longitudinally relative to the primary line of stress. Instead, in this phase of the repair process, many of the new fibers are laid down transversely, so the ability of the connective tissue they comprise to transmit force is reduced. For example, an injured Achilles tendon would be less effective at transmitting force generated by the gastrocnemius to the ankle and foot. Other damaged tissues are regenerated and new capillaries grow to provide nourishment to the new tissue during the repair phase as well.

Finally, the *remodeling phase* is consistent with increased tissue strength, though some residual pain and stiffness may remain. The collagen fibers become properly aligned, which helps restore function.

Goals of Rehabilitation and Reconditioning

The goal for treatment during the inflammatory phase is to prevent new tissue damage. A healthy diet with adequate nutrition, slow stretching that improves flexibility and encourages blood flow to the injured area, and rest are all essential for new tissue regeneration and formation. It should be noted that the strength and conditioning professional and athlete should be clear that rest is required to prevent further injury and that exercise involving the injured area is not recommended.

The goal for treatment during the repair phase is to prevent excessive muscle atrophy and joint deterioration around the injured area. Low-intensity isometric and balance exercises are indicated at this point, as strength and flexibility are usually impaired. With adequate rest, an exercise training routine that engages the muscles and tissues with the purpose of strengthening, but with minimal challenge, can help improve the injury's reparation without possibility of exacerbating the injury. It is also usually possible to do some form of conditioning exercise that does not place stress on the injured tissue, but that can maintain the athlete's fitness.

The primary goal for treatment during the remodeling phase is to optimize tissue function. Joint strengthening; exercises that prevent full range of motion, followed by exercises that allow free range of motion, and stretching and balance exercises are all recommended to be included in the athlete's exercise training program. As the athlete progresses through the remodeling phase, the modes, frequency, volume, and intensity can be adjusted to allow safe progress that coincides with the athlete's improvements.

Designing strength and conditioning programs for injured athletes requires the strength and conditioning professional to examine the rehabilitation and reconditioning goals to determine what type of program will allow the quickest return to competition without being excessively aggressive.

Following an injury, a well-designed and supervised rehabilitation and reconditioning program is important to help athletes return to action. Certain principles should be considered with this process:

- The healing tissues must never be overstressed.

- The athlete must adhere to the rehabilitative process, as outlined by the sports medicine team.

- The rehabilitation program must be evidence-based.

- The program must be individualized to the athlete and his or her specific needs and goals.

- The rehab/sports medicine team must work together to help the athlete return to unrestricted competition as quickly and safely as possible.

While an athlete is in the reconditioning period, whether it follows the competition phase or an injury, the strength and conditioning professional should be consistently aware of the intensity of workouts. Providing the athlete with a scale of 1–10 range that can communicate pain levels, the intensity, volume, and duration of workouts can be assessed and reassessed throughout the training program's progression to determine the most beneficial exercises, frequencies, and loads.

When training an athlete who is recovering from an injury, the athlete should be informed that there are two types of pain: Type I and Type II. *Type I pain* is experienced during exercise, but subsides once exercise ceases; while painful, this type of pain is not detrimental and can be recovered from within the normal recovery time periods. *Type II pain* is pain experienced 1½ hours following exercise and can last for hours or days; this pain can indicate exacerbation of the previous injury or indicate a new injury resulting from pushing too hard.

When designing a training program for athletes in the reconditioning phase, the strength and conditioning professional should start with static exercises that are pain-free and include stretching. Once flexibility improves, the program can progress through resistance exercises to increase muscle strength. As muscle strength improves, appropriate exercises that require sufficient strength and mobility can be added to the program with varying intensities, depending upon the physiological response of the athlete.

Practice Questions

1. Which of the following is a general guideline when prescribing free-weight exercises for beginners?
    a. Utilize 3 sets of 8 to 12 repetitions
    b. Utilize 5 sets of 3 to 5 repetitions
    c. Begin the training program by testing the athlete's 1RM
    d. Use new training modalities to manipulate the athlete's adaptation

2. A loading period, usually lasting 3-4 weeks of training, is termed which of the following?
    a. Macrocycle
    b. Microcycle
    c. Mesocycle
    d. Ramping cycle

3. Which of the following is a recommended intensity range for an athlete looking to increase anaerobic capacity?
    a. 67 to 75% of maximal heart rate
    b. 85 to 90% of maximal heart rate
    c. 75 to 85% of maximal heart rate
    d. 90%+ of maximal heart rate

4. What is the proper term used for muscles that oppose or support the prime mover of a movement?
    a. Agonist
    b. Synergist
    c. Secondary mover
    d. Antagonist

5. To determine the total load of a single training bout, which of the following equations should be used?
    a. Sets × repetitions
    b. Sets × repetitions x load
    c. Load × repetitions
    d. Sets × repetitions x duration

6. Which of the following is NOT considered a lower-body free-weight exercise for a beginner's program?
    a. Barbell thruster
    b. Back squat
    c. Power clean
    d. Dumbbell lunge

7. When training for power, how much rest should be given between sets?
    a. 30 seconds to 1 minute
    b. 1 to 2 minutes
    c. 3 to 5 minutes
    d. 5+ minutes

8. Which of the following terms is the principle of consistently adding resistance to an athlete's exercise in an effort to improve muscle adaptation and avoid plateaus?
    a. Progression
    b. Specificity
    c. Adaptation
    d. Overload

9. The cycle that is commonly used to prepare an athlete for more intense activity and lasts around 7 days is termed which of the following?
    a. Macrocycle
    b. Mesocycle
    c. Microcycle
    d. Preparatory cycle

10. What is the main goal for programming flexibility exercises into a training program?
    a. Warming up
    b. Cooling down
    c. Strengthening
    d. Increasing range of motion of the joints

11. Which of the following is NOT a consideration of individualized program design?
    a. Specific movement patterns of a particular sport
    b. Fatiguing exercises performed first within a training session
    c. Power movements performed first within a training session
    d. Exercise selection based around the predominant muscle fiber type used for a particular sport

12. The capability of the aerobic pathway to be activated and engaged throughout an exercise bout of a long duration is known as which of the following?
    a. Aerobic endurance
    b. Aerobic capacity
    c. Aerobic performance
    d. Anaerobic capacity

13. Proper training stance for most bilateral exercises will include which of the following body positions?
    a. Chest up, back flat, knees fully extended
    b. Straight back, heels together, knees fully extended
    c. Rounded back, soft knees, and feet shoulder-width apart
    d. Straight back, soft knees, and feet shoulder-width apart

14. Which of the following should be considered when incorporating plyometric exercises into an athlete's resistance training program?
    a. Athlete's age
    b. 1RM back squat
    c. Sex
    d. 1RM power clean

15. Which of the following training adaptations will occur when high repetitions and short rest periods are prescribed?
    a. Strength
    b. Muscular endurance
    c. Cardiovascular endurance
    d. Power

16. Why does tissue in the repair phase of injury healing lack some strength?
    a. Collagen synthesis decreases during the repair phase
    b. There are too many inflammatory cells in the area
    c. The new collagen fibers are aligned haphazardly
    d. Cellular mediators like histamine cause edema, which inhibits the function of contractile tissue

17. An exercise that is used to exhaust a single muscle group prior to performing a multi-joint exercise is known as which of the following?
    a. Pre-fatigue exercise
    b. Pre-exhaustion exercise
    c. Pre-loaded exercise
    d. Pre-failure exercise

18. Which of the following is known to promote recovery from intense bouts of exercise?
    a. Commercial energy drinks
    b. Protein supplementation
    c. Coffee
    d. Fast-paced breathing

19. Which of the following is NOT considered a basic fundamental principle for program design?
    a. Working large to small muscle groups in a workout
    b. Alternating pushing exercises with pulling exercises
    c. Alternating upper-body exercises with lower-body exercises
    d. Performing two pushes for every pull

20. Which of the following is NOT a process that occurs after an athlete sustains an injury?
    a. Inflammation phase
    b. Repair phase
    c. Rehabilitation phase
    d. Remodeling phase

21. Training sessions that include high-intensity outputs followed by short rest periods are termed which of the following?
    a. Maximum effort training
    b. Agility training
    c. Metabolic conditioning
    d. Interval training

22. What is the term used for when the body starts to return to its pre-training status after the cessation of a training program?
    a. Recovery
    b. Reversibility
    c. Atrophy
    d. Deload

23. Which of the following is NOT a mode in varying the intensity of an exercise?
    a. Utilizing slow concentric muscle actions
    b. Increasing lever length
    c. Varying balance demands
    d. Maintaining focus

24. Which of the following is considered the first proposed model of periodization, termed by Hans Selye?
    a. Linear Periodization
    b. Undulating Periodization
    c. General Adaptation Syndrome
    d. General Accumulation Syndrome

25. Which of the following rest periods should be utilized when intending to develop muscular endurance?
    a. 0 to 45 seconds
    b. 45 to 90 seconds
    c. 90 seconds to 2 minutes
    d. 2 to 5 minutes

26. The principle of the body's natural ability to grow accustomed to certain routines is known as which of the following?
    a. Accommodation
    b. Adaptation
    c. Resilience
    d. Alarm state

27. Which of the following describes a syndrome of overuse injury that occurs from irresponsible loading of intensity within a training program?
    a. Sprain
    b. Strain
    c. Microtrauma
    d. Overtraining

28. Which of the following is considered a "return to play" principle that must be taken into account when an athlete is rehabbing from an injury?
    a. The athlete should return when he or she feels able to fully participate
    b. The athlete should return when the head sport coach feels the athlete is able to participate
    c. The athlete should return when the healing tissues can be stressed without pain
    d. The athlete should return to play after completing a proper, evidence based, rehabilitation program

29. Which of the following describes minor ruptures or tears within the muscles, ligaments, and tendons that result in inhibited and limited function?
    a. Sprain
    b. Dislocation
    c. Strain
    d. Microtrauma

30. Which of the following is the correct terms that make up the *FITT Principle*?
    a. Fitness, Intensity, Training, Timing
    b. Frequency, Intensity, Time, Type
    c. Frequency, Intensity, Training, Type
    d. Fitness, Intensity, Time, Type

31. To develop power, exercises should be performed in which of the following repetition ranges?
    a. 1 to 5 repetitions
    b. 5 to 8 repetitions
    c. 8 to 12 repetitions
    d. 12 to 15 repetitions

32. Which of the following is categorized as a free-weight exercise implement?
    a. Lat pull-down machine
    b. Leg press machine
    c. Treadmill
    d. Kettlebell

33. Which of the following is considered a multi-joint exercise for the upper body?
    a. Barbell curls
    b. Triceps extensions
    c. Wrist curls
    d. Bench press

34. For the novice and intermediate athlete, which of the following training percentage ranges should be prescribed for the goal of muscular endurance?
    a. 30 to 60% of 1RM
    b. 60 to 70% of 1RM
    c. 70 to 85% of 1RM
    d. 85 to 100% of 1RM

35. The greatest resistance or weight that can be moved through the full range of motion with proper posture and in a controlled manner is known as which of the following?
    a. Maximal effort load
    b. 1 repetition maximum
    c. 1 repetition load
    d. Submaximal load

36. What does each number represent during each muscle action for an exercise with a 4×1×0 tempo?
    a. 4 second eccentric, 1 second isometric, 0 second concentric
    b. 4 second concentric, 1 second isometric, 0 second eccentric
    c. 4 second eccentric, 1 second concentric, 0 second isometric
    d. 4 second isometric, 1 second concentric, 0 second eccentric

37. When training with the main goal hypertrophy, what is the correct repetition ranges that should be prescribed?
    a. 6 to 12 repetitions
    b. 1 to 5 repetitions
    c. 12 to 20 repetitions
    d. 5 to 8 repetitions

38. The negative portion of an exercise that, when slowed down, can cause a lot of muscle damage in a minimal number of sets and repetitions is known as which of the following?
    a. Eccentric muscle action
    b. Concentric muscle action
    c. Isometric muscle action
    d. Isokinetic muscle action

39. Which of the following is the term used for the general approach to improving the fitness benefits, and reducing the incidence of injury, by systematically staggering cycles or periods of intense training?
    a. Programming
    b. Systematic intensity
    c. Periodization
    d. Long-term athletic development

Answer Explanations

1. A: Beginners should begin training by performing 3 sets of 8 to 12 reps of simple exercises using large muscle groups. This amount of total volume will allow strength adaptations, hypertrophy adaptations, and neural activations.

2. C: The mesocycle is a specific time period in periodized training intended to reach a specific goal. It is usually a 21- to 28-day training period that consists of 21 to 23 training days and five days of rest.

3. B: To increase anaerobic capacity, training intensities should remain high. Therefore, 85 to 90% of maximal heart rate should be consistently reached. To maintain a high heart rate, the training should consist of intense movements, followed by short rest periods.

4. D: An antagonist muscle is a muscle that opposes or supports the prime mover of a muscular contraction. The muscle that is involved in the contraction is known as the agonist and is considered the prime mover of the movement. The antagonist, which is the muscle involved in slowing down the contraction or resisting the movement, elongates as the agonist contracts. For every main movement of the human body, there is an agonist and an antagonist. There is also another category of musculature involved in movement: synergists. Synergists are muscles that are not directly involved with the movement but assist by stabilizing of the joints involved in the action.

5. B: Total load should be calculated to determine progressive overload and to prevent overtraining volumes. When calculating total load, the number of completed sets multiplied by the number of repetitions per set multiplied by the load used yields an accurate calculation of the total amount of weight lifted in the training session.

6. A: Lower-body free-weight training can be very beneficial to many populations, especially those within athletics. The back squat, power clean, and lunge would all be considered multi-joint, compound, lower \-body movement, whereas the barbell thruster would be more of a total body training exercise that is not commonly used for strength-gaining purposes.

7. C: Training for power should allow 3 to 5 minutes of rest between sets. This allotted time will allow the body to fully recover from the previous set so that maximal force can applied to the next set.

8. D: Overload is the principle of consistently adding resistance to an athlete's training exercises and routines in an effort to improve muscle adaptation and avoid plateaus. With the maintenance of the same resistance, muscle fibers become accustomed to the routine and fail to progress. The ideal goal is to consistently apply forces of increased weight to progress through a program to the next level of performance. With an overload of too much weight or effort, the risk of injury presents itself, so constant awareness and progressive overload should be the focus of this aspect of programming.

9. C: The microcycle is the term used for a 7-day loading period. This usually represent a week worth of training stimulus that prepares the athlete for more intense activity during the advanced stages of the training program.

10. D: Although flexibility training exercises are often utilized in warm-up sessions and cool-down sessions, the main goal of flexibility training is to increase the range of motion of the major joints of the body.

11. B: Individual considerations should include the specific movement patterns of the given sport, performing power movements first in the training session to prevent fatigue, and selecting exercises based around the predominant muscle fiber type used in the specific sport. Fatiguing exercises should not be performed first within the training session; instead, they should be performed last to prevent fatigue from reducing the technical abilities of the athlete.

12. A: Aerobic endurance refers to the capability of the aerobic metabolic pathway to be activated and engaged throughout a long exercise bout. Long-distance running, cross country skiing, endurance swimming, and triathlons are examples of sports that require highly-developed aerobic endurance.

13. D: Straight back, soft knees, and feet shoulder-width apart reflects the proper biomechanical stance for most bilateral, standing exercises. This position will allow the movement to be performed in a safe and effective manner.

14. A: The athlete's age should be considered prior to incorporating plyometric exercises into a training program. Youth, adolescents, and geriatric populations should be progressed slowly with plyometric training activities to allow the body to fully accommodate the stress that is placed on the body.

15. B: Muscular endurance will increase from high-repetition training with short rest periods. This can be very beneficial to many sports, as it allows the muscles to continually and reliably perform without premature fatigue. For example, a tennis player with good muscular endurance can stay strong, fast, and effective over a full game without seeing significant declines in swing and serve strength.

16. C: After a musculoskeletal injury, there are generally three phases of tissue healing: the inflammatory phase, the repair phase, and the remodeling phase. By the repair phase, the edema and phagocytosis from the inflammatory phase have resolved. During the repair phase, new tissue replaces the damaged tissue that has been largely removed in the inflammatory phase. Collagen synthesis increases significantly, but as the new collagen fibers aggregate at the injury site, they lay down in a haphazard manner. Instead of being aligned in the optimal arrangement (longitudinally relative to the primary line of stress), many are transversely oriented, though some are going other directions as well. This disorganization decreases the strength and functional capacity of the tissue. During the remodeling phase, the fibers assume a more "normal" and effective arrangement, which restores strength to the tissue and makes it more effective at transmitting force.

17. A: An exercise that is used to exhaust a single muscle group prior to performing a multi-joint exercise is known as pre-fatigue. Pre-fatigue is often used to increase the intensity of a training session, or to specifically target a muscle group. This technique is often used with intermediate and advanced athletes and should be used cautiously with beginners.

18. B: Whether pre- or post-training, protein supplementation has been shown to decrease recovery time after intense bouts of exercise. Other choices would hinder recovery.

19. D. Basic fundamental principles of program design include working large to small muscle groups in a workout, alternating pushing exercises with pulling exercises, and alternating upper-body exercises with lower-body exercises. Performing two pushes for every pull in the training session is not considered a fundamental principle of program design. Doing so may lead to muscle imbalances.

20. C: The rehabilitation phase is not a phase that occurs during the healing process. Instead, the three phases are the inflammation phase, the repair phase, and the remodeling phase. The inflammation phase is characterized by pain, swelling, and redness and it occurs within hours of the injury. The repair phase occurs as the number of inflammatory cells decreases and the body begins healing the injury site. Lastly, the remodeling phase is characterized by new tissue growth and strengthening of the muscles, tendons, and ligaments near the site.

21. D: Interval training includes intervals of high-intensity and low-intensity exercises throughout the workout that are alternated to maximize an athlete's cardiovascular, muscular, and overall exercise performance endurance. With consideration of an athlete's age, abilities, restrictions, and health status, an appropriate training program can be designed that implements safe intervals of high- and low-intensity exercises that maximize benefit while minimizing risk.

22. B: Reversibility is the term used for when the body starts to return to pre-training status after the cessation of a training program. When the physical stress is removed, the body responds by regressing back towards an untrained state. The result of this regression is partial or complete loss of the positive adaptations that resulted from the proper and specific training program. For strength and conditioning professionals working in high school and collegiate settings, detraining can occur during academic break periods.

23. A: Increasing lever length, varying the balance demands, and maintaining focus are all strategies to varying exercise intensity. Furthermore, all athletic activities utilize fast concentric muscle action and slowing down this portion of any exercise could hinder performance.

24. C: General Adaptation Syndrome is considered the first proposed model of periodization. Simply stated, it is the body's ability to adapt to the stress that is placed upon the body during training. Progressive overload takes general adaptation syndrome into consideration when programming for athletic development.

25. A: Adaptations in muscular endurance occur when moderate to high intensities, high volume, and short rest periods are performed. Therefore, 0 to 45 seconds would be the ideal allotted time for rest when intending to improve muscular endurance.

26. B: Adaptation is the principle of the body's natural ability to grow accustomed to certain routines. Whether it be a movement, method, mode, weight, or performance of an exercise, the body will automatically adapt to become more efficient and energy-efficient. In order to avoid adaptation in this sense, the strength and conditioning professional and athlete should work together to consistently restructure the exercises and training program to vary the muscle mechanics and gradually increase intensity and duration.

27. C: Irresponsible loading in program design can produce microtrauma. Overuse injuries are commonly seen in athletes who push the limits too much too often. Adhering to an aggressive exercise training regimen that incorporates exercises and increases in training volumes and loads is successful only if it gradually increases as an athlete's capabilities' increase and improve.

28. D: Although the athlete may feel as if he or she is ready to return, the head coach may need the athlete to participate in a competition, or the healing tissues can be stressed without pain, the athlete should not be able to compete or participate without completing a proper, evidence-based, rehabilitation program. Upon completion of this program, the body should be pain-free and the athlete should ready; these factors are still important.

29. C: Minor ruptures or tears within the muscles, ligaments, or tendons is considered a strain. While these injuries seem minimal, ruptures and tears at these specific sites can have serious ramifications and limit the ability to move and function, especially in a pain-free manner.

30. B: The FITT principle is an acronym for frequency, intensity, timing, and type—the four basic keys to designing the most beneficial training program for an athlete. With each of these factors being considered in the design of a fitness training program, the strength and conditioning professional can effectively promote an athlete's successful progression throughout the program to accommodate his or her ultimate achievement of established goals.

31. A: Power training should occur with lower repetition ranges. Therefore, exercises should be performed within the 1 to 5 repetition range. Programming low repetition ranges ensures that fatigue will stay minimal and that maximal force can be applied to each repetition.

32. D: Of the choices, kettlebells are the only implement categorized as a free-weight. Free-weights are commonly used in resistance training exercises. Including barbells, dumbbells, kettlebells, and weight plates, these pieces of equipment are convenient, transportable, and versatile in their applications for exercises targeting any major muscle group.

33. D: Barbell curls, triceps extensions, and wrist curls are all considered to be upper-body exercises. Of the potential choices, the barbell bench press is the only choice that is categorized as a multi-joint exercise for the upper body.

34. C: For novice and intermediate athletes, muscular endurance usually occurs at training percentages that fall between the 70 to 85% range.

35. C: An athlete's 1RM, or one-repetition maximum, is defined as the greatest resistance or weight that can be moved through a full range of motion with proper posture and in a controlled manner one time.

36. A: Time under tension, or TUT, is the nomenclature for each phase of the lift and is consistent with the tempo at which the exercise should be performed. Within a training set, tempo is read "eccentric—isometric—concentric" (all in seconds). Furthermore, an exercise with a 4 x 1 x 0 tempo would equate to a 4-second eccentric motion, a 1-second isometric, and an explosive concentric.

37. A: For hypertrophy-based training, the loads and volume should be high. Therefore, the athlete should perform repetitions within the 6 to 12 range to induce adaptations of muscle size and strength.

38. A: The negative or lowering portion of an exercise is an eccentric muscle action. Slow eccentrics consist of slowly lowering the weight, which can cause a lot of muscle damage in a minimal number of sets and repetitions. Reserved for advanced athletes, the recommendation is to keep sets at a load that can between 20 and 50% greater than that of 1RM. A slow eccentric usually lasts around 4 to 10 seconds and requires the strength and conditioning professional to be a spotter for assisting the athlete's concentric portion of the lift, since the weight used is greater than the athlete can handle for that portion of the lift.

39. C: Periodization is the general approach to improving the fitness benefits and reducing the incidence of injury by systematically staggering "cycles" or periods of training.

Organization and Administration

In regard to risk management in strength and conditioning, organization and administration proficiency are very important attributes for the strength and conditioning professional to possess. Having a thorough understanding of the needs of the athletes, as well as standards in the industry, will help guide the strength and conditioning professional through the process of facility design and layout. With this understanding, the strength and conditioning professional can reduce the likelihood of any legal issues that could arise from training.

Design, Layout, and Organization of the Strength and Conditioning Facility

Whether redesigning an existing facility or contributing to the design of a new facility, it is important for strength and conditioning professional to familiarize themselves with the industry standards. If the facility is already in existence when employment begins, there will be fewer modifications available and necessary, but that does not mean that the industry standards should not be met. Oftentimes, the strength and conditioning professional will be asked to design and organize a new facility for the strength and conditioning department. Following a structured design process will ensure that the facility meets industry standards. The design process includes the selection of flooring, ceiling height, mirror placement, ventilation, lighting, and equipment.

Flooring

Prior to selecting the type of flooring for the facility, it is important to ensure that the facility is on the ground floor of the building. If this option is not available, the floor should have the capacity to withstand 100 pounds per square foot. In normal circumstances, the base floor is a concrete underlayment and the top flooring consists of rubber, carpet, or turf. Wood inserts are also very common in the strength and conditioning profession, but they are primarily used for inserts within the weightlifting platforms. When determining the selection of flooring, it is important to understand the primary use for which the flooring is intended. Rubber flooring is commonly used for free weight training areas; it is very resilient, and easy to clean. Turf is an excellent selection for areas that are used for plyometric and speed training, but turf is more difficult to clean than rubber flooring. Carpet, which can be used for multiple areas, is a budget-friendly selection, but it is not as resilient as other choices, and may need to be replaced more often than the previous options.

Ceiling Height

It is important for the strength and conditioning facility to have the appropriate ceiling height for the exercises that will take place on the training floor below. Olympic exercises, plyometric training, and medicine ball exercises require a higher ceiling to allow the exercises to be performed in a safe and effective manner. The recommended ceiling height for these types of exercises is 12–14 feet. It is important to ensure that, no matter the ceiling height, there should not be any obstructions that could get in the way of the exercises being performed. Therefore, the recommended height must be clear from any low-hanging obstacles such as lights or banners.

Mirror Placement

Although mirrors are not a necessity within the strength and conditioning facility, they can be used for visual coaching and expanding the perception of the size of the facility. When utilizing mirrors, it is important to take notice of the placement of the mirror. Mirrors should be at least 20 inches from the floor. This guideline lessens the likelihood of any rolling or bouncing pieces of free-weight equipment bumping or contacting the mirror. Another guideline to note is to ensure that the mirrors are at least 6 inches away from any piece of equipment. This will give athletes, as well as strength and conditioning professionals, some room to move without coming in contact with the mirrors.

Ventilation

Ventilation is a very important aspect of the strength and conditioning facility. It is important to understand the needs of the facility when purchasing and selecting a ventilation unit. HVAC (heating, ventilation, air conditioning) selection should be based on the ability of the unit to hold a temperature during heating and air conditioning and to exchange fresh air. The temperature of the facility should be held between 68 and 78 degrees. While this temperature range is acceptable, optimal training temperatures are suggested to fall between 72 and 78 degrees. The latter temperature range allows increases the comfort of the athletes during training sessions, which enhances the quality of the training sessions.

During training sessions, staleness and humidity can arise. It is important for the strength and conditioning facility to be equipped with an HVAC system that can circulate the air. The air in the room should be replaced and exchanged 8 to 12 times per hour. Having an HVAC system that adequately accomplishes this circulation will prevent the facility from odor issues and prevent the growth of bacteria. The ventilation system should also be equipped with the ability to control the humidity of the room. The relative humidity should stay below 60 percent during all training sessions. By controlling the humidity, the comfort of the athletes during training sessions is ensured; furthermore, the risk of rust forming on the strength and conditioning equipment is minimized.

Lighting

Lighting can have a major impact in the overall feel of the facility. Many facilities are located on the outside perimeter of a building, which allows natural light to enhance the aesthetics of the room. When determining lighting for the facility, the strength and conditioning professional must ensure the room will be lit to at least 50 lumens but no more than 100 lumens. When using this guideline, the strength and conditioning professional should ensure the room is at least lit to 50 lumens when natural light is unavailable, such as during times of the day when the sun is not shining on the facility. When sunshine is entering the room, the facility should remain below 100 lumens, and it is important that the sunlight is not in the direct path of the athletes' eyesight. During this portion of the design process, the strength and conditioning professional can see why window placement becomes very important.

Equipment

When preparing the layout of the facility, certain guidelines must be met to ensure training session are run in a smooth and safe manner, and protect against any legal issues that could arise from a cluttered training area. When possible, it is recommended that equipment should be organized into groups that coincide with the goals of the training equipment. These sections could consist of a free-weight training area, an aerobic/cardio area, a stretching and warmup area, and a resistance machine area. Grouping pieces in this manner can increase the efficiency of the training sessions and provide adequate flow for athletes throughout the course of the day when multiple groups are being trained at the same times. When placing equipment, it is important to take notice of the traffic flow within the room. Many times, the designated walkways are only identified by the placement of the equipment. When designing and organizing traffic flow throughout the room, it is important to maintain at least a 36-inch walkway. This guideline will ensure that enough room is given to provide a comfortable distance away from any moving equipment.

An Example Floor Plan for a Strength and Conditioning Facility

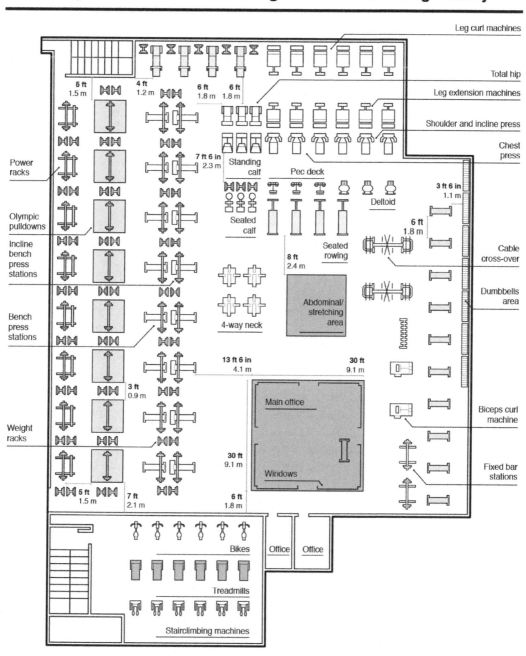

Distance Guidelines for Strength and Conditioning Facility

The following provide the recommended minimum distances that should be followed when designing the layout of the facility:

- Traffic Flow: 36–inch-wide walkways
- Warmup and Cool-Down Areas: At least 49 square feet
- Free Weight Training Area: 36 inches between ends of barbells
- Circuit Training Area: A minimum of 24 inches between machines (36 inches is the ideal space)
- Olympic Weightlifting Area: 3–4 feet between weightlifting platforms

Aerobic training equipment must be placed based on the type of equipment being used. The following provides the minimum space needed for the different pieces of cardio equipment:

- Stationary Bicycles: 24 square feet
- Treadmills: 45 square feet
- Rowers: 40 square feet
- Stair Steppers: 24 square feet
- Skiers: 6 square feet

Designing and organizing equipment with these recommendations will result in a safe and effective training facility that will be less likely to have any legal liability issues.

Primary Duties and Responsibilities of the Members of the Strength and Conditioning Staff

Obtaining an understanding of the duties and responsibilities for each strength staff member is vital to every strength and conditioning professional. By obtaining this knowledge, the strength and conditioning professional can adequately provide oversight, or assistance, for the duties and responsibilities of each staff member within the strength and conditioning department.

The head of the department is termed the Director of Strength and Conditioning or Head of Strength and Conditioning. The director has an abundant amount of responsibility in ensuring the success of the department. This person is in direct control of the operational facets such as staffing the department, overseeing all training programs, designing and maintaining the facility, complying with applicable governing bodies, and the creating the policy and procedures manual. Along with these administrative duties, the director also has direct oversight of the athletic program's physical preparedness. This position requires a vast knowledge of administrative organization and is usually offered to strength and conditioning professional.

The strength and conditioning professional's primary goal is to train athletes in physical performance, motivate athletes to push themselves to be their best, design and administer training programs that adhere to scientific foundations in strength and conditioning, and use assessment strategies to understand the needs of the athletes. With the abundant amount of responsibility for each strength and conditioning professional staff member, it is important to continually attain knowledge through continuing education in their respective organization, such as the National Strength and Conditioning Association (NSCA).

It is important that the director, as well as the strength and conditioning staff, be adequately prepared for their role in the strength and conditioning department. To begin, the strength and conditioning professional must ensure that they attain, and maintain, a professional certification. This certification should be from a nationally- and independently-accredited organization with a thorough code of ethics to ensure professionalism is properly maintained. Along with the professional certification, all strength staff members should also maintain a certification in cardiopulmonary resuscitation (CPR) and automated external defibrillation (AED) at all times.

The director of strength and conditioning may delegate responsibilities to strength staff members. These responsibilities may include facility maintenance and cleaning operations, assistance in administrative duties, and oversight of employees. Through each of these delegated responsibilities, it is important to maintain records of each performed duty. Examples of records that must be kept are personnel credentials, injury reports, staff evaluations, prior workout cards from athletic teams, and cleaning and facility maintenance checklists. These records can become essential if any legal issues arise. Records should be kept by each staff member and securely stored in a fire-secured location.

Policies and Procedures Associated with the Operation of the Strength and Conditioning Facility

Creation and adherence of a policy and procedures manual is essential for the success of the strength and conditioning department. This manual should include a mission statement, statement of program goals, program objectives, staff duties and responsibilities, operational procedures, equipment manuals, equipment cleaning duties and records, statement of return-to-participation guidelines, legal documents, and code of ethics and professionalism. Once the manual is created, it should be reviewed annually and adjusted accordingly. Another document that is often included in this manual is the *National Strength and Conditioning Association's Strength and Conditioning Professional Standards and Guidelines*.

Facility and Equipment Cleaning and Maintenance

To ensure the facility, and the equipment within the facility, is maintained and cleaned frequently enough, a checklist should be created. This checklist should include all duties related to facility and equipment upkeep, such as a schedule of when the cleaning and maintenance will be performed, floor and wall cleaning procedures, ceiling cleaning operation, and exercise equipment cleaning and maintenance requirements. This checklist should be reviewed annually, and records should be created on each date that scheduled cleaning and maintenance was performed and stored safely. These records can become vital if any legal issue arises or if an athlete is injured from a piece of equipment.

It is also important to establish a designated portion of the strength and conditioning budget for purchasing cleaning and maintenance equipment. Such equipment may include rags, towels, disinfectant, neutral floor cleaner solution, vacuum bags, and mop heads. Many instances have been reported where the strength and conditioning department did not recognize the need for this type of equipment within their budget, and subsequently, problems arose.

Facility Rules

It is very important to have compiled a rules and guideline sheet for all athletes who use the facility. By creating and enforcing all rules, the strength and conditioning professional can ensure that all training sessions are performed in a safe and effective manner. This can become very important when multiple teams are using the facility at the same time, as every athlete will have a set standard to meet in terms of facility rules. This rules document should be posted within the facility where it is easily seen and recognizable. Also, athletes and any other personnel using the facility should attend a facility orientation in which the rules are stated. Rules of the facility should include proper attire for training sessions, the preparticipation screening process, workout sheet guidelines, rules for using the equipment, the people with access to the use of the facility, and procedures involved in disciplinary actions for violations of the stated rules. It is not uncommon for strength and conditioning professionals to require signatures of all athletes who will be using the facility. This signature document should state that the athlete has read and understands all rules for the facility.

Scheduling

Specifically in high school and collegiate settings, the scheduling of training sessions can become a major obstacle that the strength and conditioning professional must overcome. Within the strength and conditioning department, it is important to state the procedures regarding how teams will be scheduled based on the time of year. Ideally, in-season teams should have priority in scheduling time at the facility because in-season teams are typically busier and have less flexible schedules. With this in mind, the strength and conditioning professional should first schedule all in-season teams based around their practice schedules, competitions, athletes' class schedules, and team meetings. It is important to have a meeting with each individual sport coach to understand the time restraints that will be placed on the athletes during the in-season schedule.

Once in-season teams are scheduled for strength and conditioning activities, the strength and conditioning professional can begin to schedule off-season teams for training sessions. When doing so, it is important to know the number of athletes on each team to ensure the supervisor to athlete ratio is being met. These ratios will be determined by the age group of the athletes, and are as follows: 1:10 for junior high school, 1:15 for high school, 1:20 for collegiate athletes. These ratios are ideal, but not always feasible. If the ratios cannot be met, the strength and conditioning professional should have a plan that works toward acquiring the correct ratio based on the age of the athletes. Oftentimes, the off-season teams will be required to train earlier in the day to provide space for the in-season teams. In educational settings, the need to split up off-season teams into multiple training sessions may be required. This can become strenuous on the strength and conditioning professional, as most of the day will be spent on training one designated team. It is encouraged to use this method sparingly to lessen the likelihood of coaching burnout.

Emergency Procedures

Having an emergency action plan is vital to the strength and conditioning professional. Neglecting to outline this type of action plan can put the athlete, facility, as well as the strength and conditioning professional at a great risk. The emergency action plan should include procedures to be followed in the event of life-threatening situations, non-life-threatening situations, and environmental situations. By designing and periodically reviewing an emergency action plan, the strength and conditioning professional can protect themselves from legal issues that could arise in an emergency event.

When designing or rewriting an emergency action plan, it is important to have all the information needed in the event of an emergency. This plan should include the emergency medical services procedures, ambulance access to the facility, location of exits, fire extinguisher locations, locations of AED equipment, telephone locations, telephone numbers for important personnel, specific location of the facility for EMS, and a procedure for each environmental situation (earthquake, tornado, fire, crime, active shooter, and terrorism). After incorporating each one of these components, it is important to share the emergency action plan with personnel beyond the strength and conditioning staff, such as medical personnel, athletic strength and conditioning professionals, administrators, and team doctors. These individuals may provide insight to overlooked aspects of the emergency action plan, or have revisions that could increase the effectiveness of the plan.

Lastly, the emergency action plan should include procedures when dealing with injuries. During the writing process of this portion of the plan, it is important to incorporate an athletic strength and conditioning professional or EMS professional. These professionals can ensure that proper procedures are conducted in the appropriate manner. Once the emergency action plan is reviewed, revised, and complete, it should be displayed in a clear and visible location. The emergency action plan should also be reviewed by the strength and conditioning staff at least once during each quarter.

Create a Safe Environment Within the Strength and Conditioning Facility

Identify Common Litigation Issues and Ways to Reduce or Minimize the Risk of Liability within the Facility

Reduction and minimization of liability issues should be a top concern for any strength and conditioning professional. Prior to addressing such issues, strength and conditioning professionals must first familiarize themselves with the terminology associated with liability.

Liability: A legal responsibility toward the athletes to ensure a safe and effective training environment, and to act accordingly in the event of injury.

Standard of Care: Refers to what a responsible strength and conditioning professional would do in the same instance if an injury would occur, or in the events leading to the injury itself.

Informed Consent: Informing the athlete of the inherent risk involved in participating in activities or procedures.

Negligence: Failure to act as a responsible strength and conditioning professional in a given emergency situation, or failing to prevent the emergency situation from happening.

When discussing the facility's liability threat, the strength and conditioning professional should be aware of six main concerns. These include preparticipation screen and medical clearance, eligibility criteria, recordkeeping, product liability, supplements, and liability insurance. Ensuring that each area is addressed is important in running a safe and effective training environment.

Preparticipation Screening and Medical Clearance
Per governing bodies, all participants of a strength and conditioning program should undergo a thorough screening process to ensure no underlying conditions are overlooked. The screening process should be performed by a healthcare provider and consist of athletic experience, past injuries, current injuries, and a physical examination. Once the screening process has taken place, the results for each individual athlete should be kept in a secure place to ensure that documents can be provided at any time.

Eligibility Criteria
Eligibility criteria refers to standards that are used to determine who is eligible to use the strength and conditioning facility. In a school environment, these individuals consist of current student-athletes, former student-athletes who have completed their playing eligibility, incoming athletes or transfers who plan to participate in an athletic sport, physical education students, athletic staff, athletic training staff, and

individuals who have been granted eligibility from the Athletic Director or Director of Strength and Conditioning. Limiting access to these groups ensures that certain criteria are met in terms of the standards of the facility and those who use it. At a public gym, the eligibility is usually open to those who have a membership or a day-pass to that gym.

Recordkeeping

Recordkeeping is vital for the strength and conditioning professional, especially in the event of injury or any legal issue that could arise. Having an organized filing system that holds preparticipation screens, medical files, injury reports, cleaning procedures and dates, manufacturer's warranties, medical waivers, and clearance forms can greatly decrease the likelihood of legal issues arising from the lack of documentation in the event of an emergency.

Product Liability

Product liability is the legal obligation of the manufacturer of products used in the strength and conditioning industry. This obligation states that the manufacturer is responsible for any injuries sustained while using the equipment. It is important for the strength and conditioning professional to review and compare manufacturers' product warranties as well as the liability statement. In reviewing these documents, the strength and conditioning professional can identify those who stand behind their products and those who do not.

Product liability will ensure that the strength and conditioning professional is unlikely to be named a main defendant when injury occurs due to the use of a piece of exercise equipment. That being said, there is still the possibility of the strength and conditioning professional being named as a codefendant, so it is important to acquire the proper liability insurance and to understand all aspects of the product liability claims. To protect themselves legally, the strength and conditioning professional should only use the manufacturer's equipment for the intended use of said equipment. Also, proper, annual maintenance should occur based on the manufacturer's recommendations and no modifications should ever be made to a piece of equipment. Finally, the strength and conditioning professional must ensure that equipment is purchased only from reputable manufacturers. Within the strength and conditioning profession, there are many companies that stand out in terms of high quality equipment. Purchasing should only occur from these companies; purchasing from low-standard companies will put the strength and conditioning professional, as well as the institution, in danger of legal issues.

Supplements

It is not uncommon for the strength and conditioning professional to be asked to recommend the use of certain supplements. They must be aware of claims of dangerous or nonresearched supplements. The strength and conditioning professional should uphold the NSCA Code of Ethics when answering questions about the use of supplements. This Code of Ethics states that the strength and conditioning professional should only recommend or provide supplementation that has undergone rigorous, long-term research and that is deemed safe and effective. It is also important to be aware of the governing bodies for which the strength and conditioning professional is working under. Many governing bodies have different rulings on the use of certain supplements, and only those that are permissible should be used.

Liability Insurance

In case any legal issue arises within the strength and conditioning industry, it is important to purchase liability insurance. The NSCA has valuable resources for acquiring such insurance and the strength and conditioning professional must take advantage in these resources. Often, the institution or gym may provide liability insurance for their strength and conditioning personnel. While this is an advantage, the strength and conditioning professional should also purchase an outside source of liability to ensure they are covered in any event. To assist in this process, strength and conditioning professionals should seek assistance from the institution's human resource manager, their legal consultant, or the resources provided by the NSCA.

Recognize Symptoms Relating to Overuse, Overtraining, and Temperature-Induced Illness

Strength and conditioning professionals are constantly stressing the human body to provide adaptations to specific demands on the body. While this is essential, it is also important to understand and recognize the symptoms of stressing the body too far. This stress can be in the form of overuse, overtraining, or stressing the body beyond its limits in extreme temperatures.

Overuse and Overtraining
Overuse and overtraining can be positive and planned within the training cycle, but they can also have detrimental symptoms if not planned accordingly. Common terms for overuse are functional overreaching and nonfunctional overreaching. Both are forms of overuse, but they have very different effects on the body in terms of long-term progress. *Functional overreaching* refers to increasing stress on the body until further stress can no longer be placed on the body without a period of recovery. This is usually planned in a period of loading stress on the athlete or athlete, followed by a period of rest, commonly referred to as a de-load period. When the load reaches a peak and is not followed by a period of de-load, stress becomes too high and detrimental consequences can occur to the athlete. If these detrimental effects occur over a significant period, the athlete may become overtrained. *Overtraining* refers to maladaptation within the training process over an extended time period, and it can take a significant amount of time to recover from. The strength and conditioning professional must be aware of the signs and symptoms of each stress category. The following will give insight to the characteristics, signs, and symptoms associated with functional overreaching, nonfunctional overreaching, and overtraining.

Functional Overreaching
Duration: Couple of days to weeks

Performance: Temporarily decreases

Signs and Symptoms:

- Short-term decrease in power production
- Short-term decrease in overall strength
- Short-term delayed onset muscle soreness
- Short-term lack of willingness or motivation to train

Nonfunctional Overreaching
Duration: Weeks to months

Performance: Decreases or stagnates

Signs and Symptoms:

- Mood disturbances and poor motivation in training
- Hormonal disturbances
- Reduced ability to recover from training sessions
- Decreased motor control
- Decreased overall strength

- Decreased overall power
- Overall increased fatigue

Overtraining
Duration: Months to years

Performance: Decreases

Signs and Symptoms:

- Emotional disturbances
- Sleep disturbances
- Increased illness and immune suppression
- Hormonal imbalances
- Anemia
- High rate of perceived exertion within training
- Loss of appetite
- Common injuries (lack of durability)
- Onset of asthma or asthma-related symptoms

Temperature-Induced Illness
Many occasions will require training in less-than-optimal training environments. Most of these such occasions will be in extreme cold or extreme heat temperatures. The strength and conditioning professional must have a thorough understanding of the signs and symptoms associated with each scenario.

Heat-Related Illness

Heat-related illness can present many signs and symptoms within the athlete. These include goose bumps, lack of perspiration, cramps, inability to speak clearly, difficulty in standing or walking, dizziness, and nausea. If the strength and conditioning professional observes any of these signs or symptoms, the activity should immediately be stopped, and the athletes should seek assistance from a medical professional or athletic strength and conditioning professional.

Heat Index *(Apparent Temperature)*

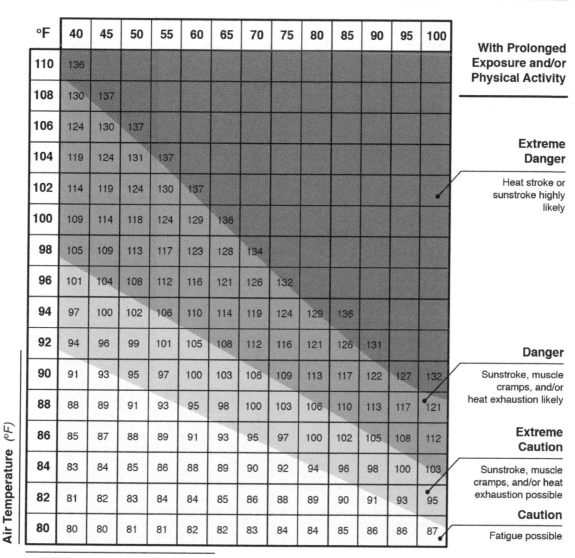

°F	40	45	50	55	60	65	70	75	80	85	90	95	100
110	136												
108	130	137											
106	124	130	137										
104	119	124	131	137									
102	114	119	124	130	137								
100	109	114	118	124	129	136							
98	105	109	113	117	123	128	134						
96	101	104	108	112	116	121	126	132					
94	97	100	102	106	110	114	119	124	129	136			
92	94	96	99	101	105	108	112	116	121	126	131		
90	91	93	95	97	100	103	106	109	113	117	122	127	132
88	88	89	91	93	95	98	100	103	106	110	113	117	121
86	85	87	88	89	91	93	95	97	100	102	105	108	112
84	83	84	85	86	88	89	90	92	94	96	98	100	103
82	81	82	83	84	84	85	86	88	89	90	91	93	95
80	80	80	81	81	82	82	83	84	84	85	86	86	87

Air Temperature *(°F)*

Relative Humidity *(%)*

With Prolonged Exposure and/or Physical Activity

Extreme Danger
Heat stroke or sunstroke highly likely

Danger
Sunstroke, muscle cramps, and/or heat exhaustion likely

Extreme Caution
Sunstroke, muscle cramps, and/or heat exhaustion possible

Caution
Fatigue possible

Cold-Related Illness

Although not as visibly observable from the strength and conditioning professional's viewpoint, effects of training in cold weather must be monitored. Signs and symptoms of cold-temperature illness include reduced heart rate, increased blood pressure, uncontrolled shivering, loss of feeling in the extremities, increased muscle tension, and decreased joint elasticity. If any of these signs are observed, the strength and conditioning professional should stop the activity and modify or move the training session to an environment where optimal temperatures are available.

Recognize When to Refer and Athlete to and/or Seek Input from Allied Health Professionals

Many instances may call for referral of an athlete or athlete to a specialized health care professional. First, the strength and conditioning professional must understand the scope of the position. Although strength and conditioning professionals oftentimes spend large amounts of time with the athlete, they must keep in mind their scope of practice. Strength and conditioning professionals are in place to increase the athlete's biological output. This can come from agility training; nutritional advice; and quickness, speed, strength, power, and balance training. When aspects of the position go beyond these areas, the strength and conditioning professional must refer the athlete to an allied health professional who specializes in the area for which the athlete needs assistance. Too often, strength and conditioning professionals try to help the athlete in areas they do not specialize in. This can place the strength and conditioning professional, the facility, or the institution in great danger of legal repercussions. Throughout the strength and conditioning professional's career, it is important to put together a team of medical professionals who can assist in such situations. Therefore, when situations beyond the scope of strength and conditioning arise with athletes, they can then be referred to a trusted medical professional who specializes in such areas. When doing so, the strength and conditioning professionals protect themselves, their facilities, and their institutions from legal issues.

The medical team should at least have a certified athletic strength and conditioning professional, a sport psychologist, a registered dietician, a physician, and a physical therapist. When all these professionals are pieced together on the same team, the athlete can benefit greatly by having a group who is solely responsible for the well-being and physical enhancement of the athlete. Within the team, each individual should recognize their roles and not provide help in areas in which other members have expertise. If an athlete is experiencing pain in the knee, he or she should be referred to an athletic strength and conditioning professional, who then can make another referral to a member on the team, if needed. While all the referrals and interactions are occurring, it is important that the entire team communicates effectively, so everyone is informed on the well-being of the athlete.

Practice Questions

1. What happens to the performance of athletes that become overtrained?
   a. It improves
   b. It declines
   c. It stays the same
   d. It improves slightly before declining

2. A legal responsibility toward the athletes to ensure a safe and effective training environment describes which legal term?
   a. Liability
   b. Tort
   c. Informed consent
   d. Negligence

3. When designing a facility, why is ceiling height important for areas of medicine ball exercises, plyometric training, and Olympic exercises?
   a. It improves the aesthetics of the facility
   b. It allows larger pieces of training equipment to be placed in the same area as the exercises being performed
   c. It ensures the exercises being performed will not be obstructed by the ceilings
   d. It allows the facility to be designed with more lighting options

4. Which of the following can safeguard against legal issues in terms of equipment liability?
   a. Modifying equipment to meet the needs of the athlete
   b. Purchasing equipment from reliable companies that stand behind their products
   c. Purchasing equipment based solely on the budget given for the project
   d. Performing maintenance on the equipment only when needed

5. Any time a facility is NOT located on the ground floor, what capacity should the floor have to withstand?
   a. 100 pounds per square foot
   b. 50 pounds per squat foot
   c. 100 pounds per square meter
   d. 50 pounds per square meter

6. To ensure training sessions are performed in a safe and effective manner, how should equipment be placed within the facility?
   a. Equipment should be organized into groups that coincide with the goals of the training equipment.
   b. Equipment should be placed in a circuit so that each different machine can be used in a high-intensity training session.
   c. Equipment should be placed around the perimeter so there is open space in the middle of the facility.
   d. Equipment should be organized depending on the amount of space each piece takes up.

7. Which of the following is NOT a sign of a heat-related illness?
    a. Cramping
    b. Inability to speak clearly
    c. Lack of perspiration
    d. Reduced heart rate

8. Why should mirrors be placed at least 20 inches from the floor?
    a. Athletes will be able to clearly see themselves in the mirror
    b. To prevent contact with any rolling or bouncing piece of free-weight equipment
    c. To give enough room for a vacuum to reach the wall without contacting the mirror
    d. To ensure athletes are in a proper position when using the mirror as a coaching tool

9. How long is the duration of nonfunctioning overreaching?
    a. Couple of hour to couple of weeks
    b. Couple of days to weeks
    c. Weeks to months
    d. Months to years

10. Which of the following is the recommended and optimal range for the temperature of the facility?
    a. 70–80 degrees recommended/72–78 degrees optimal
    b. 65–75 degrees recommended/65–72 degrees optimal
    c. 68–78 degrees recommended/68–74 degrees optimal
    d. 68–78 degrees recommended/72–78 degrees optimal

11. Why is it important to set the eligibility criteria of facility use?
    a. To ensure certain criteria are met in terms of the standards of the facility and those who use it
    b. To ensure the equipment does not become worn down from overuse
    c. To ensure participants will always have a strength and conditioning coach when training
    d. To ensure a certified medical professional is on duty at all times

12. Which of the following is NOT a main role of a strength and conditioning professional?
    a. Train athletes in physical performance
    b. Create individual nutrition plans for the athletes
    c. Motivate athletes to push themselves to be their best
    d. Design training programs that adhere to scientific foundations in strength and conditioning

13. Which of the following should NOT be included in the facility rules document?
    a. Proper attire for training
    b. Rules of using the equipment
    c. Workout sheet guidelines
    d. Emergency action plan

Answer Explanations

1. B: During times of overtraining, performance will decrease. The human body can no longer adapt to the increasing stress of the training sessions and begins to gradually decline in performance. The central nervous system will become affected and many other signs and symptoms will begin to show.

2. A: Liability is a legal responsibility toward the athletes to ensure a safe and effective training environment, as well as the ability to act accordingly in the event of injury. The other options, although legal terms, do not accurately describe the definition in the question.

3. C: Olympic exercises, plyometric training, and medicine ball exercises require a higher ceiling to allow the exercises to be performed in a safe and effective manner. Ceiling height recommendation is 12 to 14 feet for these types of exercises. It is important to ensure that the recommended height is clear from any obstructions that could get in the way of the exercises being performed. If this recommendation is not met, the training sessions may need to be altered to accommodate for the low ceiling height.

4. B: Prior to purchasing equipment, it is important to research the company and speak to those who have purchased from the company in the past. While doing research, the training and conditioning professional can easily differentiate those who stand behind their products from those who do not. All reliable companies have a thorough liability statement that explains all terms and conditions regarding the liability of their products.

5. A: Ideally, all facilities would be on the ground floor of the building. In reality, this is not always the case, and it is important to understand the flooring capacities when designing or evaluating the facility. Per recommendations, the capacity of the floor should be able to withstand 100 pounds per square foot. When complying with this recommendation, the strength and conditioning professional must ensure that the floor is strong enough to withstand the exercises being performed.

6. A: Placement of equipment is very important to the facility design process. To ensure safe and efficient training sessions, equipment should be organized into groups that coincide with the goals of the equipment.

7. D: Being able to evaluate athletes while performing exercises in extreme temperatures is a very responsibility of the strength and conditioning professional. Signs and symptoms of heat-related illnesses include goose bumps, lack of perspiration, cramps, inability to speak clearly, difficulty in standing or walking, dizziness, and nausea. Reduced heart rate is not associated with a heat-related illness, but instead is a symptom of a cold-related illness.

8. B: Although mirrors are not a necessity in the strength and conditioning facility, they are often utilized for aesthetic appeal and as a coaching tool. When designing the facility and installing the mirrors, it is recommended that the bottom of the mirrors are at least 20 inches from the floor. The main reason for this recommendation is to prevent any bumping or contact from rolling and bouncing piece of free-weight equipment, which could cause damage.

9. C: The first negative phase of overtraining is nonfunctioning overreaching. Therefore, the strength and conditioning professional must understand the signs and symptoms of overreaching, and also understand the time that may be needed to fully recover. With nonfunctioning overreaching, this recovery time ranges from weeks to months.

10. D: The recommended temperature is 68–78 degrees for the facility, while 72–78 degrees is usually considered optimal. It is important that the facility has an HVAC system that can accommodate these demands to ensure that these temperatures can be met in any situation.

11. A: Setting the standard of eligibility criteria is important for the strength and conditioning facility. Ensuring certain criteria are met in terms of the standards of the facility, and in terms of those who use it, will lessen the likelihood of legal issues, as each participant will understand the standards of the facility and be able to act accordingly.

12. B: The strength and conditioning professional has many roles for the attainment of athletic performance. That being said, when it comes to nutrition, strength and conditioning professionals must understand that they are not a registered nutritionist and therefore must refer their athletes to a registered dietician or certified nutrition professional who can create an individualized nutrition plan.

13. D: The facility rules document should outline all rules and regulations of the facility. Although an emergency action plan is a must for any strength and conditioning facility, it should be a separate document that thoroughly describes the actions in any emergency situation.

Testing and Evaluation

Testing and evaluation is vital for the strength and conditioning profession. Performing tests, as well as taking measurements, can identify athletic needs for the individual, assess the current state of the athlete, give insight on what goals to set, and evaluate the training program and rate of progress. When performing tests and measurements, it is important for the strength and conditioning professional to choose tests that are both valid and reliable for the athlete's sport. *Test validity* is the degree at which a test accurately measures what is meant to be measured for the specific athlete or sport, and *test reliability* is the degree of repeatability and consistency of a given test or measurement. Maintaining a high standard for both test validity and test reliability ensures that the tests are best suited for the given athlete or sport.

Select and Administer Tests to Maximize Test Reliability and Validity

Tests Based Upon the Unique Aspects of a Sport, Sport Position, and Training Status

When administering tests based on the specificity of one's sport, position, and training status, it is important to understand the vast array of training parameters that are conducive to optimal training within a given athletic endeavor. Therefore, test selection should be based on metabolic energy system specificity, biomechanical movement pattern specificity, experience, training status, age, sex, and environmental factors.

Metabolic Energy System Specificity
The metabolic energy system that is predominantly used within the specific sport should be considered when selecting tests that measure endurance parameters. Too often strength and conditioning professionals, as well as sport coaches, utilize endurance tests that do not accurately measure the specific energy system within the given sport. To prevent this situation, the strength and conditioning professional should acquire a thorough understanding of the specific energy demands used across multiple sports and utilize tests that measure the efficiency of the primary energy system used within the athletic endeavor.

Biomechanical Movement Pattern Specificity
Test selection should also consider important movements that are often observed within the sport and mimic these movements within the testing protocol of the athlete. Using volleyball as an example, the vertical jump test would be an appropriate test to administer because it is an important movement that is commonly used within the sport. Another area for consideration is different movements based on position within the sport. Furthermore, although the vertical jump is an important movement within the sport of volleyball, it would be more conducive for the outside hitters than for the liberos on the team. Therefore, the liberos may require a separate test to accurately measure their performance within their position.

Experience and Training Status
For a given test to be considered reliable and valid, the test must also be selected based on the previous experience and training status of the athlete. If technical proficiency is not yet met for a given exercise, using that exercise as a test would void the reliability and validity of that test. Therefore, the strength and conditioning professional should choose exercises that the athletes have shown to be proficient at. Furthermore, training status must also be considered during the test selection process. Any test that is not

conducive to the specific demands of the sport should not be tested in late offseason, early preseason, or late preseason as the athlete should be training toward the specific demands of the sport, rather than the specific demands of the test.

Age and Sex

Age and sex should also be considered when selecting tests for athletes. Younger-aged athletes will have a difficult time performing the same distances as adolescent and college-age athletes when performing aerobic capacity tests. Furthermore, young athletes may have not developed the strength or technique required for valid and reliable strength-based testing. Therefore, the strength and conditioning professional must ensure that the testing is age-appropriate, to ensure reliability and validity of the test. The sex of the athlete will also play a role in the type of testing performed. One main concern is the relative strength difference between males and females. Males typically have a higher relative strength within athletics. Therefore, using a maximum repetition chin-up test may be conducive to the male athletes, but female athletes may have a harder time achieving accurate results. Instead, the strength and conditioning professional could administer a maximum repetition chin-up test with the male athletes and a maximum prone pull-up test, with the feet elevated, for the female athletes. This modification would ensure accurate, valid, and reliable testing results for each group of athletes.

Environmental Factors

Environmental factors must be considered to ensure test validity and reliability. Temperature, humidity, altitude, and running surfaces can all alter testing results. Therefore, when available, the strength and conditioning professional should utilize environmentally-controlled indoor facilities, especially when aerobic endurance tests are being performed. If indoor facilities are not available, strength and conditioning professionals should use their professional judgment on whether the environment will affect the testing results. If they conclude that the environment will affect the testing results, a different test may be warranted to ensure the results are reliable and valid.

Test Administration Procedures That Use Equipment, Personnel, and Time Efficiently

Test administration procedures are vital to the outcome of testing results. Ensuring the tests are administered in an organized manner can enhance athlete safety, as well as ensure the testing results accurately portray the current training status of the athlete. Therefore, the strength and conditioning professional must ensure that the tests are well organized and administered, appropriate testers should be carefully trained, and athletes should be properly instructed. Each of the following points will ensure that tests are performed in a safe, reliable, and organized manner:

Health and Safety Considerations

Although all participants should be medically cleared with a complete physical examination, the strength and conditioning professional must be aware of the current health of all athletes. Testing often places athletes in stressful situations that require maximal output and exertion, and such situations can worsen preexisting conditions or present new ones. Therefore, the strength and conditioning professional must be very cognizant of the health status of all athletes before, during, and after any testing that requires maximal output from the participants. Athletes should be allowed water and breaks as much as personally needed between maximal bouts of exertion to further increase the validity of the tests and ensure dehydration or fatigue does not cause any unreliable test results. Furthermore, throughout testing, attendance of medical personnel and athletic training staff may be warranted to further increase the health and safety of the athletes.

Selecting and training testing personnel is equally as important as the tests that are selected. Ensuring that all testers are qualified and knowledgeable in each test is vital to the validity and reliability of testing results. Once selected, all testers should undergo an educational session in which each test is explained and witnessed. Throughout this educational session, explanation of testing parameters should be thoroughly explained to ensure consistency with all testers. Furthermore, test administrators should develop a checklist for all test administrators that incudes materials required for each test and written test sheets with answers to common questions that might arise during the testing session.

Along with the selection and training of testers, the strength and conditioning professional, as the main administrator of the test, should develop recording forms and sheets for each test administrator. This form or sheet should have a place for each result for each participant of the test. Developing these sheets will ensure that the testing will be run efficiently and in an organized manner and that no results fall through the cracks.

When possible, athletes should be tested by one tester. Allowing one tester to test each participant will eliminate the possibility of poor interrater reliability confounding the results. *Interrater reliability* refers to how reliable test results are when different raters observe and score the test. There is often a decrease in the reliability of the test due to multiple testers, as the judgement standard could slightly change dependent on the individual who is administering the test. If this is not possible due to the number of athletes being tested at once, the strength and conditioning professional should select tests that have a well-defined or objective judging process, such as a push-up test where depth of the push-up is standardized or a timed mile run.

Vertical Jump Test

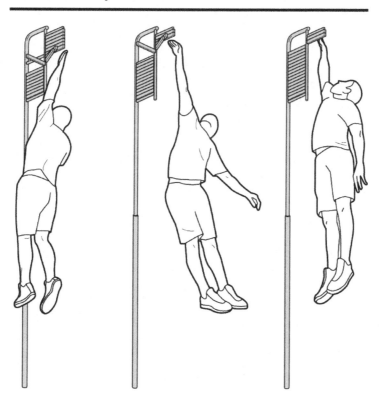

Sequence of Tests

The sequence of the tests being performed is vital to the validity and reliability of the testing results. A complex understanding of exercise science and proper testing sequencing is paramount in ensuring that the testing results are accurate. With the energy systems and proper work-to-rest ratios being accounted for, the strength and conditioning professional should perform high-skill testing and non-fatiguing tests prior to those of requiring less skill and that induce more fatigue. The following provides some basic guidelines to follow when creating the test sequence. The tests are listed in the order in which they should be administered:

- Non-fatiguing tests such as height, weight, skinfold, mobility, and vertical jump
- Agility tests that allow participants maximal recovery time should follow the non-fatiguing tests
- Maximum power tests such as the 1RM Power Clean or 1RM Snatch
- Maximum lower body strength tests such as the 1RM Squat
- Maximum upper body strength tests such as the 1RM Bench
- Sprint testing
- Local muscular endurance testing
- Fatiguing anaerobic capacity tests
- Aerobic capacity tests

By following the test sequencing guidelines, the strength and conditioning professional can ensure that the performance in one test will not adversely affect the reliability and validity of the results of subsequent tests.

Preparing Athletes for Testing

Prior to test day, athletes should be aware of what tests they are to perform so they can physically and mentally prepare. In the week, or weeks, prior to the test, explanation of each test should be well-demonstrated and athletes should be allowed to ask questions about the test.

On test day, the strength and conditioning professional should perform a thorough warmup with each participant. The warmup should consist of a general warmup to increase body temperature and joint mobility, followed by a specific warmup that is geared toward the testing that will be performed for that day. By administering a thorough warmup, the strength and conditioning professional ensures that athletes' results will provide validity and reliability to the test battery.

Administer Testing Protocols and Procedures to Ensure Reliable Data Collection

Testing Equipment and Its Proper Use

For the strength and conditioning professional, using proper testing equipment and using it correctly, is very important in ensuring that accurate data are collected. Most equipment used within testing is equipment that is often found in most strength and conditioning facilities: power racks, barbells, weight plates, cones, measuring tapes, and stopwatches. While these pieces of equipment are vital to most testing, it is very important to ensure that each one is well-maintained, so that it can handle the maximal loads that are often observed in 1RM testing. With most weight-oriented testing, the same guidelines that are used in training are observed in testing: proper form from participant, proper spotting from coaches and participants, proper instruction, and proper supervision.

When using cones and other location markers, placement is vital. Proper placement of cones, at the proper distances, will ensure that the testing is valid and reliable. Stopwatches should be well-maintained and batteries should be changed every 3–6 months to ensure correct functioning during testing periods. Measurement equipment should be properly placed and secured to ensure that the equipment does not move during the testing session.

Specific testing may require the use of specialized equipment. Skinfold calipers, bodyweight scales, and height measurement tools are often used within testing to attain body composition measurements, as well as to record anthropometry results. Each of these specialized pieces of equipment should be purchased with literature explaining the proper use within testing. Each member of the testing staff should read and understanding the literature to ensure the piece is being used properly and with accurate precision. Again, validity and reliability are vital when acquiring testing data; therefore, all pieces of testing equipment should be well-maintained and used properly.

Testing Procedures

Proper procedures for testing are very specific to the testing battery. To begin, the strength and conditioning professional must ensure that all participants undergo a proper warmup prior to testing. The warmup should include a general session to increase blood flow and core temperature. The general warmup session should be followed by a specific warmup to prepare the body for the specific testing that is to follow. Once the participants have undergone the warmups, the tests should begin. Following the sequence of tests, the participants will begin the testing battery with the first test. During testing, coaching cues should be continuous, and encouragement should be given to each individual athlete. Oftentimes, athletes will begin to encourage each other during the testing process. Although this is positive, the strength and conditioning professional must ensure that the testing participant does not become distracted by the overwhelming encouragement and is still able to focus on the test. Once all participants have performed the first test, subsequent tests will follow.

For maximum strength tests, the athlete should be allowed to "work up" in weight. It would not be advantageous to allow the athlete to begin the test at a maximal weight, as the nervous system would not be ready for such weight. Therefore, a proper allotted time for warmup sets should precede the 1RM testing. The following will provide guidelines to use when performing 1RM testing for maximum strength tests:

1RM Testing Protocol
Athletes are instructed to begin with a light resistance that allows 5–10 repetitions followed by a 1–minute rest period.

The strength and conditioning professional will then estimate a warmup load that the athlete will perform for 3–5 repetitions. A 10- to 20-pound increase is suggested for upper-body exercises and 30–40-pound increases are suggested for lower-body exercises.

The second set will be followed by a 2–minute rest period.

Next, the strength and conditioning professional will estimate a near-maximal load that will allow the athlete to perform 2–3 repetitions. Another 10–20 pound (or 5%–10%) increase is suggested for upper-body exercises and a 30–40 pound (or 10%–20%) increase is suggested for lower-body exercises.

The third set will be followed by a 2-4-minute rest period.

The strength and conditioning professional will continue to make load increases for 1 repetition until near maximal loads are reached.

2–4-minute rest periods should be allowed between near-maximal attempts.

The process will continue until the athlete performs a successful maximal attempt with proper form. Ideally, this process will take the athlete 3–5 sets to obtain a valid and reliable 1 repetition maximum.

Work-to-Rest Ratios

When performing the test battery, work-to-rest ratios should be followed closely to ensure fatigue does not dictate the testing results. Testing work-to-rest ratios should follow the needs of the energy system that is primarily being used or tested within the testing session. For phosphagen-based tests, the work-to-rest ratio should be 1:12–1:20. Fast glycolysis-based tests will require less time in between bouts of exertion; therefore, the work-to-rest ratio should be within 1:3–1:5. Oxidative-based tests should require a 1:1–1:3 work-to-rest ratio. It is important to understand that these guidelines are for typical athletes, and more time may be needed if the athlete is displaying fatigue during the test or between the exertion bouts of the test.

Testing to Assess Physical Characteristics and Evaluate Performance

As previously stated, specific tests will be conducive to certain athletes and specific sports. It is important for the strength and conditioning profession to acquire knowledge in specific to the needs of the sport or individual. The following will provide tests that are commonly used in the attainment of specific data based on the specific needs of the athlete:

Maximum Muscular Strength (Low-Speed Strength)
- 1RM Bench Press
- 1RM Bench Pull
- 1RM Back Squat

Although these tests are considered maximum strength tests, the bar speed will be slower than those of other maximum strength tests. If maximum strength (in power) is to be measured, the following tests should be performed:

Maximum Muscular Power (High-Speed Strength)
- 1RM Power Clean
- Standing Long Jump
- Vertical Jump
- Static Vertical Jump
- Reactive Strength Index
- Margaria-Kalaman Test

Anaerobic Capacity
- 300–Yard Shuttle (274 Meters)

Local Muscular Endurance
- Partial Curl-Up
- Push-Up
- YMCA Bench Press Test

Aerobic Capacity
- 1.5 Mile Run (2.4 km)
- 12-Minute Run
- Yo-Yo Intermittent Recovery Test
- Maximal Aerobic Speed Test

Agility
- T-Test
- Hexagon Test
- Pro Agility Test
- 505 Agility Test

Speed
- Straight-Line Sprint Test

Balance and Stability
- Balance Error Scoring System (BESS)
- Star Excursion Balance Test (SEBT)

Flexibility
- Sit-and-Reach Test
- Overhead Squat

Anthropometry
- Girth Measurements

Body Composition
- Skinfold Measurements

An Example of a Subscapular Skinfold Measurement

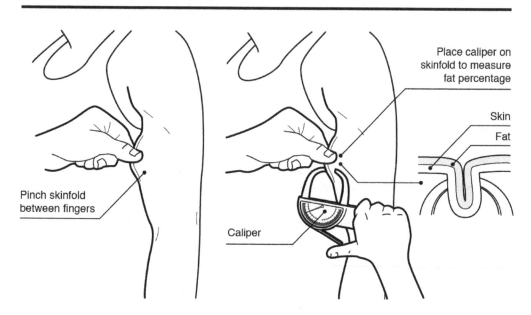

Pinch skinfold between fingers

Place caliper on skinfold to measure fat percentage

Skin

Fat

Caliper

To provide valid and reliable testing results, the strength and conditioning professional should be well-rehearsed in each of the previous tests, as a vast majority of sports will require a selection of these tests to develop a well-designed test battery.

Evaluate and Interpret Test Results

Once the testing sessions are complete and all the data have been collected, the strength and conditioning professional can begin analyzing, evaluating, and interpreting the testing results. This data collection will give insight on the analysis of an individual athlete's performance profile, analysis of a team based on previous team's testing data, or analysis of relative data compared to typical test results observed within the specific sport. The following sections provide information on the types of analysis used within the strength and conditioning profession.

Validity of Test Results

As previously stated, validity refers to the degree to which a test measures what it is intended to measure. Ensuring valid tests were performed, proving post-test validity is very important to show the testing was accurate for the given athlete or sport. To ensure validity, the strength and conditioning professional should utilize a multistep analysis: Did the test battery measure what it was intended to measure? How efficiently were the tests performed? Did the test battery follow the proper guidelines to ensure validity? Were the athletes properly prepared for the tests? To enhance future testing, emphasis must be placed on the evaluation of the testing process and the changes that may be needed to enhance the process. Furthermore, the strength and conditioning professional should acquire knowledge in the specific areas of validity to further establish the general validity within the test battery. Specific validity types consist of face validity, construct validity, criterion-referenced validity, and content validity.

Face Validity
Face validity relates to the perception of the athlete or a casual observer of whether the selected test accurately measures what it is intended to measure. It is sort of a subjective confirmation that a test "appears" to measure what it is designed to measure. Within strength and conditioning testing sessions, face validity can greatly enhance or confound the testing results. Athletes tend to try harder and perform better on tests with higher face validity, such as the vertical jump test, as they believe in the validity and utility of the test. If, at any time, the strength and conditioning professional believes an athlete doesn't perceive the test to have merit, they should thoroughly explain the test and how the data received from such test provide insight on the performance of the athlete or athletes. By doing so, the face validity of the given test should be enhanced.

Construct Validity
Construct validity is the basis of all validity measures used for testing. Furthermore, *construct validity* is the ability of a test to portray the underlying construct. To be considered a valid test, the test should pertain to the specific sport, the specific movement patterns of the given sport, appear meaningful, have meaningful utility based on individual athletes, include a number of trials to allow for error, permit appropriate scoring, and be able to withstand the scrutiny of statistical evaluation. By checking each one of these aspects, the strength and conditioning professional can ensure that the test battery was well-established, valid, and repeatable.

Criterion-Referenced Validity

Criterion-referenced validity refers to the extent to which test scores can be associated with other tests that measure the same athletic ability. There are three subcategories within criterion-referenced validity: concurrent validity, convergent validity, and predictive validity.

Concurrent validity refers to the extent to which the test scores are comparable with the test scores of different tests for the same ability. An example would be the use of a jump pad, which measures vertical jump height, compared to the use of a Vertec, which measures the same ability. Although a jump pad is widely accepted as a way to measure the vertical jump height of an athlete, often the accuracy is not believed to be the same as that of a Vertec.

Convergent validity refers to the extent to which the test correlates with the testing data of the "gold standard" test used for the given athletic ability. Using the vertical jump measurement again, the Vertec would be considered the gold standard. How well the jump pad measurement correlates with the data received from the Vertec would be considered convergent validity. Convergent validity is often used within the strength and conditioning profession when explaining the reasoning behind a certain selection of a given test. Oftentimes the use of more efficient testing, the need for fewer testing personnel, and the need for using less equipment are considered when determining the convergent validity over the gold standard test.

Predicative validity refers to the extent to which the test battery can be used to predict success within a given athletic endeavor or sporting event. Predictive validity measures the performance of given tests and corresponds the testing data with the success of the sport.

Content Validity

Content validity refers to the extent to which the tests correlate with a given athlete or sport, under the assessment of an expert. Content validity is much like face validity, but where face validity is the perception of a general observer or athlete, content validity is the perception of an expert within the field of strength and conditioning.

Typical Versus Atypical Test Results Based on a Sport or Sport Position

Once validity has been established, the strength and conditioning professional can begin to compare the normative results of the test battery to the typical results observed within the sport, position, or population. By doing so, insight will be attained on specific performance parameters as they pertain to a certain individual or sport team.

Further analysis should be performed to begin developing insight based on the typical test results often observed within the given sport or athlete. The National Strength and Conditioning Association provides information on typical results observed with a vast majority of sporting activities. Such information includes percentile values for the 1RM bench press, 1RM back squat, 1RM power clean, vertical jump heights, body weight and composition, and bench pull. This typical data is also sorted by sport and position and information is provided for sports such as men's and women's soccer, men's and women's basketball, American football, baseball, and volleyball. Further testing data can also be found in the National Strength and Conditioning database, as well as in the *Journal of Strength and Conditioning Research*. By comparing the results from the test battery to those often observed within the given sport or athlete, the strength and conditioning professional can identify specific areas that need to be improved upon in future training programs, and also what specific needs are being met with the current training program.

Design or Modification of the Training Program Based on Test Results

Once validity has been established and proper analysis has taken place based on the testing results, the strength and conditioning professional should begin adjusting the training program of the individual athlete or specific sport. Submaximal results will often require some adjustments within the training program to further enhance the physical capabilities of the athlete. When designing or modifying elements the program, the strength and conditioning professional should follow basic programming guidelines to ensure proper periodization is followed for the new stressor within the training program.

In most cases, based on testing data, program modifications will be the result of a submaximal performance within the testing battery. Lower-body strength, upper-body strength, and total body power are often key indicators for which modifications will be required for optimal performance. Furthermore, designing and developing an athletic profile for each athlete can track long-term progress throughout the training process. This athletic profile can highlight the main capabilities of each athlete, as well as body composition statistics throughout a multiyear training program.

It is important to note that not all training programs will require modifications based on the testing data. Modifications and changes to the training program should only be performed when a significant capability is not being met with optimal results. One flaw that is common within the strength and conditioning profession is changing the program too soon without allowing time for proper adaptation to occur with a given capability. Steadily allowing progress within the specific capabilities required for a given sport will have the most impact on the optimal performance of the individual athlete.

Practice Questions

1. Which of the following is NOT a subcategory of criterion-referenced validity?
    a. Concurrent validity
    b. Convergent validity
    c. Predictive validity
    d. Construct validity

2. To measure endurance parameters for a specific individual athlete or sport, which of the following can ensure validity and reliability?
    a. Use testing protocols that are specific to the energy demands of the athlete
    b. Ensure athletes are using maximal effort
    c. Require minimal rest between bouts
    d. Use an aerobic-based test regardless of individual or sport

3. To begin 1RM testing, which of the following should occur first?
    a. Athletes should start with a load of 70% of the goal 1RM.
    b. Athlete should begin with a light resistance for 5–10 repetitions.
    c. Athletes should start with a load of 80% of the goal 1RM.
    d. Athletes should begin with a light resistance for 1–3 repetitions.

4. Which of the following athletic capability is tested by the Yo-Yo Intermittent Recovery Test?
    a. Local muscular endurance
    b. Agility
    c. Aerobic capacity
    d. Anaerobic capacity

5. Which of the following is NOT used during body composition and anthropometry testing?
    a. Skinfold calipers
    b. Stopwatch
    c. Bodyweight scale
    d. Height measurement tools

6. Which of the following could lessen the validity and reliability of a given test?
    a. Using exercises where technical proficiency has yet to be met
    b. Using exercises that the athletes are accustomed to
    c. Using exercises the are specific to the biomechanical movement patterns of the sport
    d. Using exercises that are specific to the sex of the athlete

7. Which of the following reflects the proper work-to-rest ratio for oxidative-based testing protocols?
    a. 1:12–1:20
    b. 1:5–1:10
    c. 1:1–1:3
    d. 1:3–1:5

8. Why is it important to compare the final testing data with the typical testing data associated with the specific sport or individual athlete?
   a. To show that the current program is effective
   b. To show the sport coaches that the strength and conditioning coach is competent
   c. To prove content validity
   d. To depict specific athletic capabilities that need to be improved upon

9. Which of the following will help to ensure the health and safety of the athlete during a testing session?
   a. Athletes should be allowed water and breaks, at will
   b. Athletes should be encouraged to push themselves to maximal intensity at all times
   c. Rest periods should push the limits within the work-to-rest ratios
   d. Only the testing administrator should be present during testing sessions

10. Which of the following is considered a maximum muscle power testing protocol at high speeds?
    a. 1RM back squat
    b. 1RM deadlift
    c. 1RM power clean
    d. Maximum push-up

11. Which of the following describes a common flaw that occurs after analyzing testing data?
    a. Not making any modification to the current training program
    b. Completely changing the entire periodization of the program
    c. Punishing athletes based on the testing results
    d. Changing the program without giving ample time for proper adaptation to occur

12. For valid and reliable testing results, which of the following should be FIRST within the sequence of testing protocols?
    a. Maximum lower body tests
    b. Maximum power tests
    c. Maximum upper body tests
    d. Local muscular endurance tests

13. Which of the following is NOT an acceptable test for maximum muscular strength with low speeds?
    a. 1RM bench press
    b. 1RM back squat
    c. 1RM partial curl-up
    d. 1RM bench pull

14. Skinfold calipers are commonly used for which of the following measurements?
    a. Body mass index (BMI)
    b. Girth measurements
    c. Anthropometry
    d. Body composition

15. To optimally prepare athletes for testing, which of the following should occur?
    a. Testing sessions should not be known to the athletes prior to testing
    b. Athletes should be made aware of what tests they are to perform
    c. The test day should be known but the specific tests should not
    d. The tests should be explained but the testing day should not be known

16. Which of the following is NOT a consideration of environmental factors within testing sessions?
    a. Athlete's clothing
    b. Humidity
    c. Temperature
    d. Running surface

17. How many testing personnel are encouraged for optimal, valid data during testing sessions?
    a. One tester to enhance the validity of the testing data
    b. Two testers per athlete
    c. Multiple testers for optimal testing efficiency
    d. Athletes can be used for testing personnel to enhance the availability of personnel used for testing sessions

18. To ensure optimal preparation, which of the following should occur prior to testing within the testing session?
    a. Athletes should perform maximal power testing upon arrival to the testing location.
    b. A proper warmup should occur to increase core temperature and joint elasticity.
    c. Athletes should undergo endurance testing upon arrival to the testing location.
    d. A proper warmup should occur to decrease core temperature and joint elasticity.

19. Ideally, how many testing sets should be performed to measure the 1RM data?
    a. 1–2 testing sets
    b. 1–3 testing sets
    c. 3–5 testing sets
    d. 5–8 testing sets

20. The perception of the athlete, or casual observer, of whether the selected test accurately measures what it is intended to measure describes which of the following validity types?
    a. Construct validity
    b. Content validity
    c. Criterion-referenced validity
    d. Face validity

Answer Explanations

1. D: Although construct validity is a category within general validity, it is not a subcategory of criterion-referenced validity and is separate from the other options. Criterion-referenced validity refers to the extent to which test scores can be associated with other tests that measure the same athletic ability. Within criterion-referenced validity are three subcategories: concurrent validity, convergent validity, and predictive validity.

2. A: The metabolic energy system that is predominantly used within the specific sport or position should be considered when selecting tests that measure endurance parameters. By utilizing testing protocols that are specific to the energy demands of the athlete, the strength and conditioning professional can ensure the validity and reliability of the administered testing protocols.

3. B: To ensure accurate and valid testing results, it is important for the strength and conditioning professional to acquire a thorough understanding of proper procedures when administering 1RM testing. By following the guidelines within the 1RM testing protocol, the strength and conditioning professional should instruct the athlete to warm up with a light resistance that easily allows 5–10 repetitions.

4. C: The Yo-Yo Intermittent Recovery Test measures the aerobic capacity of the athlete. This test is widely used across many sports, especially when an accurate measurement of the athlete's aerobic capacity is desired.

5. B: Body composition and anthropometric testing often use skinfold calipers, bodyweight scales, and height measurement tools. Although stopwatches are used for many testing protocols, they are not used for body composition or anthropometric testing protocols.

6. A: For a given test to be considered reliable and valid, the test must also be selected based on the previous experience and training status of the athlete. If technical proficiency is not yet met for a given exercise, using that exercise as a test would void the reliability and validity of that test. Therefore, the strength and conditioning professional should choose exercises that the athletes have shown to be proficient at.

7. C: Acquiring a thorough understanding of the proper work-to-rest ratios is vital for the testing to be considered valid and reliable. For oxidative-based testing protocols, a 1:1–1:3 work-to-rest ratio should be used.

8. D: The function of such a comparison is to identify specific athletic capabilities that need to be improved upon. Once validity has been established, the strength and conditioning professional can begin to compare the normative results of the test battery to the typical results observed within the sport, position, or population. By doing so, insight will be attained on specific performance parameters as they pertain to an individual or sports team. Furthermore, by comparing the results from the test battery to those often observed in the given sport or athlete, the strength and conditioning professional can depict specific areas that need to be improved upon in future training programs.

9. A: To help support the health and safety of the athletes, athletes should be allowed water and breaks as often as personally needed between maximal bouts of exertion. Allowing water breaks increases the validity of the test and ensures dehydration or fatigue does not cause any unreliable test results. It also keeps athletes safe.

10. C: Although the 1RM back squat and deadlift are considered maximum power tests, they are considered low-speed tests. Therefore, the 1RM power clean is the only option that coincides with a maximum high-speed power test. A maximum push-up test would be considered a local muscular endurance test.

11. D: Not all training programs will require modifications based on the testing data. Modifications and changes to the training program should only be performed when a significant capability is not being met with the current program. One flaw that is common within the strength and conditioning profession is changing the program too soon without allowing time for proper adaptation to occur with a given capability.

12. B: With the energy systems and proper work-to-rest ratios being accounted for, the strength and conditioning professional should perform high-skill testing and non-fatiguing tests prior to those requiring less skill and are more fatiguing. Therefore, within the given options, maximum power tests should be performed first, due to the other options being less skill-dependent and more fatiguing in nature.

13. C: Although the partial curl-up is commonly used within many testing batteries in the strength and conditioning profession, it is not tested with a 1RM format. Instead, the partial curl-up is used for local muscular endurance testing. Other options such as the 1RM bench press, back squat, and bench pull are commonly used for testing maximum muscular strength at low speeds.

14. D: The only acceptable option for the use of skinfold calipers is body composition. Body mass index, girth measurements, and anthropometric testing require the use of other specialized testing equipment.

15. B: Prior to test day, athletes should be aware of what tests they are to perform so they can physically and mentally prepare. In the days or week prior to the test, the strength and conditioning professional should fully explain each test and athletes should be allowed to ask questions about the test.

16. A: Although the appropriate clothing is important for accurate and valid testing results, it is not a consideration that falls within the environmental factors of the testing session. Instead, consideration should be given to the specific environmental factors of temperature, humidity, and running surface.

17. A: Selecting and training testing personnel is equally as important as the tests that are chosen. Ensuring that all test administrators are qualified and knowledgeable in each test is vital to the validity and reliability of testing results. When possible, athletes should be tested by one tester to reduce the possibility of poor interrater reliability confounding thee results.

18. B: On test day, the strength and conditioning professional should make sure all participants engage in a thorough warmup. The warmup should consist of a general warmup to increase body temperature and joint elasticity, followed by a specific warmup that is geared toward the testing that will be performed that day.

19. C: Following the guidelines set forth by the National Strength and Conditioning Association, 3–5 testing sets are ideal when performing 1RM testing. The 3–5 sets will ensure the athletes are given enough attempts, while also preventing fatigue within the testing session.

20. D: Face validity relates to the subjective perception, usually from the athlete, of whether the selected test accurately measures what it is intended to measure. Athletes tend to try harder and perform better on tests with higher face validity, as they believe in the validity and utility of the test.

Greetings!

First, we would like to give a huge "thank you" for choosing us and this study guide for your CSCS exam. We hope that it will lead you to success on this exam and for your years to come.

Our team has tried to make your preparations as thorough as possible by covering all of the topics you should be expected to know. In addition, our writers attempted to create practice questions identical to what you will see on the day of your actual test. We have also included many test-taking strategies to help you learn the material, maintain the knowledge, and take the test with confidence.

We strive for excellence in our products, and if you have any comments or concerns over the quality of something in this study guide, please send us an email so that we may improve.

As you continue forward in life, we would like to remain alongside you with other books and study guides in our library. We are continually producing and updating study guides in several different subjects. If you are looking for something in particular, all of our products are available on Amazon. You may also send us an email!

Sincerely,
APEX Test Prep
info@apexprep.com

FREE

Free Study Tips DVD

In addition to the tips and content in this guide, we have created a FREE DVD with helpful study tips to further assist your exam preparation. **This FREE Study Tips DVD provides you with top-notch tips to conquer your exam and reach your goals.**

Our simple request in exchange for the strategy-packed DVD is that you email us your feedback about our study guide. We would love to hear what you thought about the guide, and we welcome any and all feedback—positive, negative, or neutral. It is our #1 goal to provide you with top quality products and customer service.

To receive your **FREE Study Tips DVD**, email freedvd@apexprep.com. Please put "FREE DVD" in the subject line and put the following in the email:

a. The name of the study guide you purchased.

b. Your rating of the study guide on a scale of 1-5, with 5 being the highest score.

c. Any thoughts or feedback about your study guide.

d. Your first and last name and your mailing address, so we know where to send your free DVD!

Thank you!

Made in the USA
Middletown, DE
22 December 2018